PSYCHIATRIC ASPECTS OF SYMPTOM MANAGEMENT IN CANCER PATIENTS

Edited by

William Breitbart, M.D.

Psychiatry Service and Pain Service
Memorial Sloan-Kettering Cancer Center
Department of Psychiatry
Cornell University Medical College
New York, New York

Jimmie C. Holland, M.D.

Psychiatry Service
Memorial Sloan-Kettering Cancer Center
Department of Psychiatry
Cornell University Medical College
New York, New York

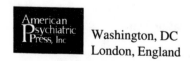

Washington, DC
London, England

Copyright © 1993 American Psychiatric Press, Inc.
ALL RIGHTS RESERVED
Manufactured in the United States of America on acid-free paper.
First Edition   96 95 94 93 4 3 2 1

American Psychiatric Press, Inc.
1400 K Street, N.W., Washington, DC 20005

Library of Congress Cataloging-in-Publication Data

Psychiatric aspects of symptom management in cancer patients / edited
    by William Breitbart, Jimmie C. Holland. — 1st ed.
        p.   cm. — (Clinical practice ; no. 25)
    Includes bibliographical references and index.
    ISBN 0-88048-193-5 (alk. paper)
    1. Cancer—Psychological aspects.   2. Cancer—Palliative
    treatment.   3. Cancer—Patients—Mental health.   4. Psychiatry.
I. Breitbart, William, 1951–   .   II. Holland, Jimmie C., 1928–
    III. Series.
        [DNLM: 1. Neoplasms—psychology.   2. Neoplasms—therapy.
3. Palliative Treatment.   W1 CL767J no. 25]
RC262.P782   1992
616.99′4′0019—dc20
DNLM/DLC
for Library of Congress   92-6969
                                                                CIP

British Library Cataloguing in Publication Data

A CIP record is available from the British Library.

For my parents, Rose and Morris Breitbart, my wife Rachel, my son Samuel Benjamin, and in memory of my uncle Henry Breitbart.

Contents

Contributors

Michael A. Andrykowski, Ph.D.
Assistant Professor, Department of Behavioral Science, University of Kentucky College of Medicine, Lexington, Kentucky

William Breitbart, M.D.
Assistant Professor, Department of Psychiatry, Cornell University Medical College; Assistant Attending Psychiatrist, Psychiatry Service, Pain Service, Department of Neurology, Memorial Sloan-Kettering Cancer Center, New York, New York

Harvey Max Chochinov, M.D., F.R.C.P.C.
Assistant Professor of Psychiatry, Department of Psychiatry, University of Manitoba; Psychiatric Consultant, Manitoba Cancer Center Treatment and Research Foundation, Winnipeg, Manitoba, Canada

Stewart B. Fleishman, M.D.
Clinical Assistant Professor of Psychiatry, Albert Einstein College of Medicine; Attending Psychiatrist, Division of Psychiatric Oncology, Long Island Jewish Medical Center, New York, New York

Kenneth Gorfinkle, Ph.D.
Assistant Professional in Psychiatry, Columbia University College of Physicians and Surgeons; Clinical Psychologist, Behavioral Medicine Program, Department of Psychiatry, Presbyterian Hospital, New York, New York

Jimmie C. Holland, M.D.
Professor, Department of Psychiatry, Cornell University Medical College; Chief, Psychiatry Service, Wayne E. Chapman Chair in Psychiatric Oncology, Memorial Sloan-Kettering Cancer Center, New York, New York

Sharon A. Horowitz, A.C.S.W.
Research Social Worker, Pain Service, Department of Neurology,
Memorial Sloan-Kettering Cancer Center, New York, New York

Paul B. Jacobsen, Ph.D.
Assistant Professor of Psychiatry, Department of Psychiatry, Cornell
University Medical College; Assistant Attending Psychologist,
Psychiatry Service, Department of Neurology, Memorial
Sloan-Kettering Cancer Center, New York, New York

Kathryn M. Kash, Ph.D.
Instructor of Psychology in Psychiatry, Department of Psychiatry,
Cornell University Medical College; Clinical Assistant Attending
Psychologist, Psychiatry Service, Department of Neurology, Memorial
Sloan-Kettering Cancer Center, New York, New York

Lynna M. Lesko, M.D., Ph.D.
Associate Professor, Department of Psychiatry, Cornell University
Medical College; Associate Attending Psychiatrist, Psychiatry Service,
Department of Neurology, Memorial Sloan-Kettering Cancer Center,
New York, New York

Jon A. Levenson, M.D.
Assistant Clinical Professor of Psychiatry, Department of Psychiatry,
College of Physicians and Surgeons, Columbia University; Assistant
Attending Psychiatrist, Department of Psychiatry, Presbyterian
Hospital, New York, New York

Mary Jane Massie, M.D.
Associate Professor, Department of Psychiatry, Cornell University
Medical College; Associate Attending Psychiatrist, Psychiatry Service,
Department of Neurology, Memorial Sloan-Kettering Cancer Center,
New York, New York

Steven D. Passik, Ph.D.
Instructor, Department of Psychiatry, Cornell University Medical
College; Clinical Assistant Psychologist, Psychiatry Service,
Department of Neurology, Memorial Sloan-Kettering Cancer Center,
New York, New York

William H. Redd, Ph.D.
Professor, Department of Psychiatry, Cornell University Medical College; Attending Psychologist, Psychiatry Service, Department of Neurology, Memorial Sloan-Kettering Cancer Center, New York, New York

Elisabeth J. Shakin, M.D.
Instructor, Department of Psychiatry and Human Behavior, Thomas Jefferson University Hospital, Jefferson Medical College, Philadelphia, Pennsylvania

Introduction
to the Clinical Practice Series

*O*ver the years of its existence the series of monographs entitled *Clinical Insights* gradually became focused on providing current, factual, and theoretical material of interest to the clinician working outside of a hospital setting. To reflect this orientation, the name of the Series has been changed to *Clinical Practice*.

The Clinical Practice Series will provide books that give the mental health clinician a practical, clinical approach to a variety of psychiatric problems. These books will provide up-to-date literature reviews and emphasize the most recent treatment methods. Thus, the publications in the Series will interest clinicians working both in psychiatry and in the other mental health professions.

Each year a number of books will be published dealing with all aspects of clinical practice. In addition, from time to time when appropriate, the publications may be revised and updated. Thus, the Series will provide quick access to relevant and important areas of psychiatric practice. Some books in the Series will be authored by a person considered to be an expert in that particular area; others will be edited by such an expert, who will also draw together other knowledgeable authors to produce a comprehensive overview of that topic.

Some of the books in the Clinical Practice Series will have their foundation in presentations at an annual meeting of the American Psychiatric Association. All will contain the most recently available information on the subjects discussed. Theoretical and scientific data will be applied to clinical situations, and case illustrations will be utilized in order to make the material even more relevant for the practitioner. Thus, the Clinical Practice Series should provide educational reading in a compact format especially designed for the mental health clinician–psychiatrist.

Judith H. Gold, M.D., F.R.C.P.C.
Series Editor
Clinical Practice Series

Clinical Practice Series Titles

Family Approaches in Treatment of Eating Disorders (#15)
Edited by D. Blake Woodside, M.D., M.Sc., F.R.C.P.C., and
Lorie Shekter-Wolfson, M.S.W., C.S.W.

Adolescent Psychotherapy (#16)
Edited by Marcia Slomowitz, M.D.

Benzodiazepines in Clinical Practice: Risks and Benefits (#17)
Edited by Peter P. Roy-Byrne, M.D., and Deborah S. Cowley, M.D.

Current Treatments of Obsessive-Compulsive Disorder (#18)
Edited by Michele Tortora Pato, M.D., and Joseph Zohar, M.D.

Children and AIDS (#19)
Edited by Margaret L. Stuber, M.D.

Special Problems in Managing Eating Disorders (#20)
Edited by Joel Yager, M.D., Harry E. Gwirtsman, M.D., and
Carole K. Edelstein, M.D.

Suicide and Clinical Practice (#21)
Edited by Douglas Jacobs, M.D.

Anxiety Disorders in Children and Adolescents (#22)
By Syed Arshad Husain, M.D., F.R.C.P.C., F.R.C.Psych., and
Javad Kashani, M.D.

Psychopharmacological Treatment Complications in the Elderly (#23)
Edited by Charles A. Shamoian, M.D., Ph.D.

Responding to Disaster: A Guide for Mental Health Professionals (#24)
Edited by Linda S. Austin, M.D.

Psychiatric Aspects of Symptom Management in Cancer Patients (#25)
Edited by William Breitbart, M.D., and Jimmie C. Holland, M.D.

**Madness and Loss of Motherhood: Sexuality, Reproduction, and
Long-Term Mental Illness (#26)**
Edited by Roberta J. Apfel, M.D., M.P.H., and Maryellen H. Handel, Ph.D.

Treatment of Adult Survivors of Incest (#27)
Edited by Patricia L. Paddison, M.D.

**Rediscovering Childhood Trauma: Historical Casebook and Clinical
Applications (#28)**
Edited by Jean M. Goodwin, M.D., M.P.H.

Introduction

Symptom Control and Quality of Life: Role of the Psychiatrist in the Oncology Setting

*O*ver the past decade increasing attention has been given to the quality of life of patients undergoing treatment for cancer. There is a growing awareness that quality of life is of importance from the time of cancer diagnosis through treatment and into the terminal phases of illness. This trend has been due to a number of factors, including increased survival of patients with cancer, the growth of medical consumerism, the backlash against overly aggressive and technological interventions, the rise of the hospice movement and the discipline of palliative medicine, and the growth of behavioral medicine and health psychology. For cancer patients, quality of life is highly dependent on the alleviation of distressing physical and psychological symptoms. Symptom control in cancer patients was initially left primarily to medical physicians and oncologists who focused on physical symptoms.

The oncological and palliative care literature reflects the explosion of interest and research in areas such as antiemetic therapies for postchemotherapy nausea and vomiting, the use of opioids in managing cancer pain, and the applications of hormonal therapies in the treatment of cancer-related cachexia. The entrance of psychiatrists and psychologists into the oncology setting has broadened the concept of symptom control to include the diagnosis and treatment of psychological symptoms such as anxiety, depression, and confusion, as well as behavioral (conditioned) symptoms such as anticipatory nausea and vomiting, anorexia, and phobias. An appreciation of the interaction of psychological and physical symptoms has led to the development of multidisciplinary approaches to the management of symptoms in cancer patients.

This book grew out of a symposium entitled "Psychiatric Symptom Control in Cancer Patients," which was presented at the annual meeting of the American Psychiatric Association in Montreal in May 1988. As in the symposium, there are two general themes in this text: 1) the management of psychiatric complications of cancer and 2) the psychiatric and psychological management of physical symptoms in cancer patients. The purpose of this book is to present to psychiatrists and other mental health professionals working in the oncology setting a comprehensive and practical resource for the management of symptoms of both a psychological and physical nature. The contributors to this volume have been chosen for their unique ability to bring a combination of clinical and research experience to the review of these problems. They represent faculty of the Memorial Sloan-Kettering Cancer Center Psychiatry and Pain Services, as well as colleagues who have had close association with these two groups. Their disciplines include psychiatry, psychology, and social work. This diversity has made this volume quite accessible to a wide range of clinicians providing care to cancer patients.

The authors of the first two chapters address the management of the common psychiatric syndromes encountered in the oncology setting. In Chapter 1, Massie and Shakin review the management of depression and anxiety in the cancer patient. In Chapter 2, Fleishman, Lesko, and Breitbart describe the spectrum of organic mental disorders seen in cancer patients and provide strategies for their management. Both chapters use extensive case examples and present useful pharmacological and psychotherapeutic interventions.

The authors of the next seven chapters focus on psychiatric and behavioral approaches to physical symptom control. Breitbart and Passik present a review of psychiatric aspects of cancer pain management in Chapter 3, including useful cognitive behavioral interventions, as well as an extensive review of the use of psychotropic drugs as adjuvant analgesics. In Chapter 4, Lesko addresses the problem of eating disorders in the cancer setting, including the assessment and management of anorexia, cachexia, and food aversions using pharmacological and behavioral approaches.

Andrykowski and Jacobsen provide an extensive review of the problem of anticipatory nausea and vomiting associated with cancer chemotherapy in Chapter 5. This common problem represents a paradigm for the behavioral control of cancer treatment related symptoms.

In Chapter 6, Gorfinkle and Redd discuss behavioral interventions in the pediatric population and review the behavioral control of anxiety, distress, and learned aversions in children receiving cancer treatment.

In Chapter 7, Horowitz and Breitbart provide a practical guide to the use of common behavioral interventions such as relaxation and imagery. Scripts for the application of these techniques are included as helpful examples for the novice wishing to employ behavioral techniques. Breitbart, Levenson, and Passik address the special symptom control needs of terminally ill cancer patients in Chapter 8. The authors extensively review the assessment and management of symptoms such as pain, nausea, dyspnea, constipation, and other common problems of the terminally ill that impact on quality of life.

Chochinov discusses the management of grief in the cancer setting in Chapter 9. He addresses the issues of loss and anticipatory bereavement and distinguishes between normal and pathological manifestations of grief. Finally, in Chapter 10, Kash and Breitbart conclude with an overview of countertransference issues as they relate to psychiatric work with cancer patients and an update on the stress of work in the oncology setting experienced by doctors and nurses. The authors also outline a role for psychiatric involvement in staff stress interventions.

As mental health professionals become increasingly involved in the care of patients with chronic diseases, such as cancer, there is a growing need for us to become more familiar with the palliative aspects of treatment. An integration of psychological and physical dimensions of care is essential to enhanced comfort, well-being, and quality of life in cancer patients. Attention to these aspects of symptom control are often, unfortunately, limited to the end stages of illness. This book is meant to serve as a guide to the enhancement of our patients' lives, through control of their distressing symptoms, throughout the course of illness.

We wish to thank and acknowledge all of the authors who contributed to this book, the members of the Psychiatry Service of Memorial Sloan-Kettering Cancer Center, our patients, and our families. John Blanchette provided valuable assistance in preparation of the manuscripts for this book and we thank and acknowledge his dedicated work.

William Breitbart, M.D.
Jimmie C. Holland, M.D.

Chapter 1

Management of Depression and Anxiety in Cancer Patients

Mary Jane Massie, M.D.
Elisabeth J. Shakin, M.D.

*P*atients show remarkable resilience in their ability to adapt to both the diagnosis and the treatment of cancer. Understandably, patients who are diagnosed as having cancer react with significant levels of emotional distress. The fears and uncertainties associated with the diagnosis—possible death, pain, disfigurement, disability, and disrupted relationships—are similar in most people. When the stress related to the diagnosis and treatment of cancer is severe or persistent, or when patients' emotional resources are insufficient to cope with the stress, psychological distress may result. When distress interferes with cancer patients' ability to participate in their treatment or to function adaptively, psychiatric evaluation may be warranted to evaluate the clinical significance of anxiety and depression. "Anxiety" and "depression" are, therefore, not surprisingly, the most common reasons for referral of patients in oncology settings (Massie and Holland 1989).

Prevalence of Psychiatric Disorders Among Cancer Patients

In 1983, Derogatis et al. reported the prevalence of psychiatric disorders among 215 randomly accessed hospitalized and ambulatory cancer patients. Using DSM-III criteria (American Psychiatric Association 1980), slightly more than half (53%) of the patients evaluated were adjusting normally to stress. However, 47% of the patients met DSM-III criteria for a psychiatric disorder. Of these, more than two-thirds (68%) had reactive anxiety or depression (adjustment disorders with depressed or anxious mood); 13% had a major depression; 8% had an organic mental disorder; 7% had a personality disorder; and 4% had preexisting anxiety disorders. Approximately 85% of those patients with a psychiatric disorder had depression or anxiety as the central symptom. More than half of the patients evaluated by the Psychiatry Service at Memorial Sloan-Kettering Cancer Center are diagnosed as having adjustment disorders, often with mixed features of anxiety and depression; major depression is diagnosed in 10% of patients and anxiety disorders in 4% (Massie and Holland 1987a).

Depression

Sadness is an expected emotional reaction at the time of diagnosis of cancer and at key points during its course, especially during advanced stages. It is important to be able to distinguish between "normal" degrees of sadness and "abnormal" levels of depression in cancer patients. Recognition of pathological levels of depression for which psychiatric consultation is needed and for which treatment should be instituted is a critical aspect of patient care (Massie 1989a, 1989b).

Prevalence of Depression

The prevalence of depression in the general population has been estimated to be 6% (Locke and Reiger 1985). Thus only a small number of cancer patients can be expected to have a preexisting affective disorder that places them at increased risk of depression during the course of cancer. The frequency of depression among cancer patients has been the subject of numerous studies; the reported rates have ranged from as high as 58% (Hinton 1972) to as low as 4.5% (Lansky et al. 1985). The highest frequency of depression is reported in studies that depend on clinician reports of depressive symptoms with absence of defined diagnostic criteria for depression and in studies that assessed patients with more advanced stages of disease and more severe levels of illness (i.e., hospitalized patients [Bukberg et al. 1984]).

In the past, depression was thought to be greater in patients with cancer than in those with other medical illnesses. Estimates of the frequency of depression in hospitalized cancer patients, many with advanced disease, has ranged from 20% to 25% (Plumb and Holland [1977] estimated 20% to 23%, Bukberg et al. [1984] 24%, and Koenig et al. [1967] 25%). Similar prevalence rates of depression have been found among patients on general medical floors (Moffic and Paykel 1975; Schwab et al. 1967), suggesting that cancer patients may not be more depressed than other equally ill medical patients (Plumb and Holland 1977).

Vulnerability to Depression

With data from studies in extensive clinical observations, it is now possible to predict which patients are at highest risk for depression. The factors that increase the risk of depression are history of affective disorder or alcoholism, advanced stage of cancer, increased physical impairment, pancreatic cancer, poorly controlled pain, and treatment with medications or concurrent illnesses that produce depressive symptoms (Holland et al. 1986; Shakin and Holland 1988). When specific organic factors can be identified as causes of depression, organic mood syndrome should be considered as the diagnosis.

Numerous commonly prescribed medications can produce symptoms of depression: α-methyldopa, reserpine, barbiturates, diazepam, steroids, and propranolol ("Drugs That Cause" 1989). Of the more than 285 cancer chemotherapeutic agents now available, depressive symptoms are produced by relatively few: vincristine, vinblastine, procarbazine, L-asparaginase, amphotericin B, and interferon ("Cancer Chemotherapy" 1987; "Drugs of Choice" 1991). The glucocorticoids prednisone and dexamethasone are widely used as critical components of many standard treatments and can cause psychiatric disturbances, ranging from minor mood disturbances to steroid psychosis (Stiefel et al. 1989). Mood changes resulting from steroids include a sense of well-being, emotional lability, euphoria, and/or depression, sometimes with suicidal ideation.

Many metabolic, nutritional, endocrine, and neurological disorders produce symptoms that can be mistaken for depression. Cancer patients with abnormal serum levels of potassium, sodium, or calcium may appear depressed, as can patients who are febrile, anemic, or deficient in vitamin B_{12} and folate. Hyper- or hypothyroidism, Cushing's syndrome, hyperparathyroidism, and adrenal insufficiency must be considered in the differential diagnosis of the depressed cancer patient; if they are present, appropriate treatment should be instituted. Finally, depression is also a common sequela of chronic pain syndromes; adequate pain control must first be established before a diagnosis of major depressive disorder can be established.

Clinical Picture

The normal response to hearing the diagnosis of cancer is sadness about the loss of health and anticipated losses, including death. This normal response is part of a spectrum of depressive symptoms that range from normal sadness to adjustment disorder with depressed mood to major depression. Symptoms are minimal when stresses are few, but may become severe when a crisis occurs.

The clinical evaluation includes a careful assessment of symptoms, mental status, physical status, treatment effects, and laboratory data. The clinician should obtain information about previous depressive episodes and substance abuse, any family history of depression or suicide, concurrent life stresses, and the availability of social support. The disease-related symptoms of anorexia, fatigue, weight loss, and insomnia in patients with cancer cannot be distinguished from the neurovegetative symptoms of depression in medically healthy patients. The diagnosis of depression in the cancer patient must, therefore, rest on the presence of other symptoms: dysphoric mood or appearance, crying, anhedonia, decreased self-esteem, guilt, feelings of hopelessness and helplessness, and suicidal ideation (Breitbart and Holland 1988; Massie and Holland 1987b). Depression in cancer patients is best evaluated by assessing the severity of dysphoric mood; the feelings of hopelessness, guilt, and worthlessness; and/or the presence of suicidal thoughts.

Suicidal ideation always requires careful assessment to determine whether the talk of suicide is a patient's way of exerting ultimate control over intolerable symptoms or whether talk of suicide is a prelude to suicidal acts. Suicide may occur in the context of a major depression, adjustment disorder, delirium, or organic mood syndrome. Although suicidal ideation is common in cancer patients, relatively few patients act on these impulses. Nowadays, most depressed cancer patients are treated as outpatients or are treated on medical oncology units. It is rare that transfer to a psychiatric unit is necessary or feasible.

Breitbart (1987, 1989) outlined factors that place a cancer patient at a high risk of suicide: poor prognosis and advanced illness, depression and hopelessness, uncontrolled pain, delirium, prior psychiatric history, history of previous suicide attempts or family history of suicide, history of recent death of friends or spouse, history of alcohol abuse, and few social supports. Often the suicide attempts in our hospital have occurred either in a patient with poorly controlled pain, a mild encephalopathy, and disinhibition secondary to medications or in a patient who was both hopeless and distressed about being unable to communicate his or her discomfort to caregivers.

Management of Depression in Cancer Patients

The cornerstone of good management of depressed cancer patients is the consistent emotional support given by the oncologist and the treatment team. Oncologists are encouraged to consider psychiatric consultation when patients' depressive symptoms have lasted longer than a week, when they are worsening rather than improving, and when they are interfering with the patients' ability to cooperate with treatment. Short-term psychotherapy with crisis intervention is a useful mode of psychotherapy in these patients.

Psychotherapy

The goals of psychotherapy are to help patients regain their sense of self-worth, to correct misconceptions about the past and present, and to integrate the present illness into a continuum of life experiences. The therapist should emphasize past strengths and support previously successful ways of coping. This helps patients mobilize inner resources as they move ahead, modifying plans for the future and accepting necessary limitations.

Both the patient and the family often perceive the depressive symptoms as evidence that the cancer patient has "given up." Family members and the patient need to hear the psychiatrist explain the biological (if present) and psychological influences contributing to the depressed mood, the proposed interventions, and the anticipated timing of response to treatment.

The number of psychotherapy sessions is obviously highly variable; however, 4–10 sessions are usually sufficient to reduce symptoms to a tolerable level. Prolonged and severe depression usually requires treatment that combines psychotherapy with somatic treatment, either medication or electroconvulsive therapy. If suicidal risk is present in a hospitalized cancer patient, 24-hour nursing companions should be used to monitor suicidal thinking and to provide continued observation and support for the patient. The following case illustrates the treatment of an elderly depressed cancer patient who expressed suicidal thoughts:

Case 1

Ms. A, a 67-year-old woman with breast cancer metastatic to her bones and lungs, was admitted for management of shortness of breath related to pleural effusions. Chest tubes were inserted and sclerosis was performed; however, she complained of severe chest pain. She became depressed and tearful and voiced concern that pain meant that her death was near. She stated that she no longer wished to live. Ms. A's inpatient management included a 24-hour companion, pain control (hydromorphone hydrochloride [Dilaudid] 4 mg every 4 hours around the clock), and amitriptyline (50 mg at bedtime). She responded well and was ultimately transferred to a hospice where she was able to have unrestricted visits with her grandchildren. Ms. A remained pain free and in generally good spirits until her death 2 months later.

Pharmacotherapy

The antidepressants most commonly used for cancer patients (Table 1–1) are the tricyclic antidepressants (TCAs). TCAs are started in low doses (10–25 mg at bedtime) and are increased slowly over days to weeks, until symptoms improve. Cancer patients generally require lower total therapeutic doses (25–125 mg po) than does a medically healthy depressed patient (150–300 mg po). The choice of a particular agent depends on the side effect profile of the TCA, a history of response to specific agents, and the nature of the patient's medical and depressive symptoms. Amitriptyline and doxepin are preferred in agitated, depressed patients with insomnia when sedation is desired. Desipramine and nortriptyline are less sedating and are preferable in patients who are more sensitive to anticholinergic side effects (e.g., patients with brain metastases). Antidepressants with significant anticholinergic side effects should be avoided in patients with decreased intestinal motility, stomatitis, or urinary retention. Because patients taking multiple medications with anticholinergic side effects (e.g., analgesics and neuroleptics) may be at increased risk for anticholinergic delirium, the least anticholinergic antidepressants should be prescribed. Most TCAs can be prepared as rectal suppositories for patients who are unable to take oral medications or who are unable to receive injections (because of low platelet counts). Amitriptyline, imipramine, and doxepin can be given intramuscularly if the patient is unable to take oral medication ("Drugs That Cause" 1989).

If a patient does not respond to a TCA, or cannot tolerate its side effects, an atypical antidepressant (e.g., bupropion, fluoxetine,

Table 1–1. Antidepressant medications used in treating cancer patients

Drug name (by class)	Starting daily dosage (mg po)	Therapeutic daily dosage (mg po)
Tricyclic antidepressants		
Amitriptyline	25	75–100
Doxepin	25	75–100
Imipramine	25	75–100
Desipramine	25	75–100
Nortriptyline	25	50–100
Atypical antidepressants		
Bupropion	15	200–450
Fluoxetine	20	20–60
Trazodone	50	150–200
Sertraline	50	50–150
Heterocyclic antidepressants		
Maprotiline	25	50–75
Amoxapine	25	100–150
Monoamine oxidase inhibitors		
Isocarboxazid	10	20–40
Phenelzine	15	30–60
Tranylcypromine	10	20–40
Lithium carbonate	300	600–1200
Psychostimulants		
Dextroamphetamine	2.5[a]	5–30
Methylphenidate	2.5[a]	5–30
Pemoline	18.75[a]	37.5–150
Triazolobenzodiazepines		
Alprazolam	0.25–1.00	0.75–6.00

[a]At 8 A.M. and noon.

trazodone, and sertraline) or a heterocyclic antidepressant (e.g., maprotiline and amoxapine) can be used. Atypical antidepressants are generally considered to be less cardiotoxic than are TCAs (Glassman 1984). Bupropion is a relatively new drug in the United States, and we do not have much experience with its use in medically ill patients. At present, it is not the first drug of choice for depressed patients with cancer; however, we would consider prescribing bupropion if patients have a poor response to a reasonable trial of other antidepressants. Bupropion may be somewhat activating in medically ill patients; it should be avoided in patients with seizure disorders and brain tumors and in those who are malnourished.

Trazodone is strongly sedating and in low doses (100 mg at bedtime) is helpful in the treatment of depressed cancer patients with insomnia. Effective antidepressant dosages are often greater than 300 mg per day. Trazodone is highly serotonergic; its use should be considered when patients require adjuvant analgesic effect in addition to antidepressant effects (France 1987). Trazodone has been associated with priapism and should, therefore, be used with caution in male patients.

Fluoxetine, a selective inhibitor of neuronal serotonin uptake, has fewer sedative and autonomic effects than the TCAs (Cooper 1988). The most common side effects are mild nausea and a brief period of increased anxiety. Fluoxetine can cause appetite suppression usually lasting for a period of several weeks. Some of our patients have experienced transient weight loss, but weight usually returns to baseline levels. The anorectic properties of fluoxetine have not been a limiting factor in our use of this drug in cancer patients. In general, the side effect profile of fluoxetine may make it a more favorable treatment for depressed medically ill patients.

The heterocyclic antidepressants have side effect profiles that are similar to those of the TCAs. Maprotiline should be avoided in patients who are at high risk for seizures because the incidence of seizures can be increased with this medication. Amoxapine has strong dopamine-blocking activity; hence, patients who are taking other dopamine blockers (e.g., antiemetics) have an increased risk of developing extrapyramidal symptoms and dyskinesias.

A history of response to a monoamine oxidase inhibitor (MAOI) may make these agents a logical choice for the depressed cancer patient. The actual use of MAOIs, however, is generally less well received because they impose further dietary restrictions on the patient who may already have nutritional deficiencies and dietary restrictions related to cancer. MAOIs are absolutely contraindicated in patients receiving meperidine and should be used cautiously in patients receiving other narcotics because of hypertensive reactions. Sympathomimetics and the chemotherapeutic agent procarbazine (also an MAOI) can cause hypertensive crises when used in combination with an MAOI.

The psychostimulants—dextroamphetamine, methylphenidate, and pemoline—promote a sense of well-being, decrease fatigue, and stimulate appetite at low doses in cancer patients (Fernandez et al. 1987). Treatment with dextroamphetamine and methylphenidate is usually initiated at a dose of 2.5 mg at 8:00 A.M. and noon. The advantage of these drugs is their rapid onset of antidepressant action compared with that of the TCAs. Typically, patients are maintained on methylphenidate for 1–2 months and approximately two-thirds will be able to be withdrawn from methylphenidate at the time without a recurrence of depressive symptoms. Patients who develop recurrence of depressive symptoms can be maintained on methylphenidate for long periods of time (e.g., up to 1 year) without evidence of significant abuse. Tolerance will develop and adjustment of the dose may be necessary.

Pemoline, a less potent psychostimulant, (Chiarello and Cole 1987) comes in a chewable tablet so patients who have difficulty swallowing can absorb the drug through the buccal mucosa. We have begun to use pemoline frequently in a population of cancer patients with depressive symptoms and it appears to be as effective as methylphenidate and dextroamphetamine. Pemoline should be used with caution in patients with renal impairment, and liver function tests should be monitored periodically with longer-term treatment. Psychostimulants can potentiate the analgesic effects of narcotic analgesics, while at the same time counteracting unwanted daytime sedation (Bruera et al. 1989). Occasionally psychostimulants can produce nightmares, insomnia, and even psychosis.

The triazolobenzodiazepine alprazolam is effective in treating both anxiety and depression in cancer patients. Treatment is initiated with dosages of 0.25 mg tid and titrated up to effective antidepressant doses, usually from 4 to 6 mg per day. Abrupt discontinuation of alprazolam can result in seizures.

Electroconvulsive Therapy

Occasionally (but rarely), electroconvulsive therapy (ECT) is given to depressed cancer patients. As in medically healthy patients, ECT is used for the treatment of delusional and severe endogenous depressions. Depressed cancer patients for whom ECT should be considered are those with life-threatening depressions, those who have responded well to ECT in the past, those who are unable to tolerate the effects of antidepressants, and/or those who have not responded to antidepressants. Such patients may present with refusal to eat, mutism, or severe suicidal ideation. The only absolute contraindication to ECT is increased intracranial pressure. Space-occupying lesions in the brain and recent myocardial infarction are only relative contraindications.

Anxiety

The types of anxiety most frequently encountered in cancer patients are outlined in Table 1–2. They include reactive anxiety (adjustment disorder with anxious mood), anxiety related to a preexisting anxiety disorder that is exacerbated by medical illness (panic disorder, phobias, generalized anxiety disorder [GAD], and posttraumatic stress disorder [PTSD]), and anxiety related to physical illness (organic anxiety syndrome).

Reactive Anxiety

By far, the most common type of anxiety seen in cancer patients is *reactive anxiety,* which corresponds to adjustment disorder with anxious mood in DSM-III-R (American Psychiatric Association 1987). It is the task of the clinician to distinguish the normal fear generated by the diagnosis of cancer and its treatment from the anxiety of an adjustment disorder. Almost all patients experience some anxiety on days before routine follow-up visits to their oncologist or after completion of lengthy cancer treatments (e.g., radiation) (Holland et al. 1979; Scott 1983). Patients who first learn of a cancer diagnosis or of a recurrence of disease often experience a period of initial shock and turmoil, irritability, and disruption of sleep and appetite. The ability to concentrate and carry out usual life patterns is impaired and patients experience intrusive thoughts about the diagnosis as well as fears of the future. Other crisis points include waiting for the start of any new treatment (e.g., surgery, radiotherapy, and chemotherapy), waiting for test results, a change in treatment after learning of relapse, the anniversary of illness-related events, and the advanced or terminal stages of illness. The impaired ability to concentrate and carry out usual life patterns usually resolves gradually over 1 to 2 weeks, particularly if patients receive support from their family, friends, and physician.

The distinction between an adjustment disorder and the normal fear generated by the cancer diagnosis is based on duration and intensity of symptoms, as well as on degree of functional impairment. Often we encounter cancer patients whose anxiety is so high that it interferes with their compliance with the cancer treatment. Social and familial interactions become impossible. For such patients, the long duration of various treatments and the recurrent nature of the disease itself may prolong the duration and intensity of maladaptive reactions. Uncertainty about the future and treatment effectiveness is a common theme in anxious cancer patients. In advanced stages of disease, patients fear the death process, anticipating increasing physical disability and uncontrolled pain and suffering.

Anxiety Related to a Preexisting Anxiety Disorder

Panic disorders, phobias, GAD, and PTSD are distinguished from the other anxiety disorders as being long-lasting, often antedating the

Table 1–2.   Types of anxiety in cancer patients

Reactive anxiety
    Adjustment disorder with anxious mood
    Adjustment disorder with mixed emotional features
Preexisting anxiety disorders
    Panic disorder
    Phobias
    Generalized anxiety disorder
    Posttraumatic stress disorder
Anxiety related to medical illness
    Uncontrolled pain
    Metabolic causes
    Medication side effects
    Withdrawal states
    Hormone-producing tumors

cancer diagnosis. They are characterized by the extreme fear of losing control and of being overwhelmed by various circumstances. The exacerbation of these anxiety disorders can interfere with the patient's ability to cooperate with cancer treatments, and management of these anxiety disorders becomes imperative (Massie 1989a).

Panic disorder occurs with or without agoraphobia and consists of unexpected, sudden anxiety attacks that are accompanied by shortness of breath, paresthesias, chest pain, palpitations, nausea, and fear of dying. The treatment of panic attacks in a patient with cancer requires careful attention to the patient's overall medical and personal situation. Reactivation of the symptoms of panic disorder may occur in the cancer setting. Patients can be treated with the triazolobenzodiazepine alprazolam, TCAs, and MAOIs. Propranolol is useful in blocking the autonomic manifestations of panic. The following case example illustrates the usefulness of combining treatments for panic attacks in a patient with cancer:

Case 2

Ms. B, a 27-year-old professional, was referred for evaluation of anxiety and depression after resection of a liposarcoma from her left thigh. She was started in weekly psychotherapy, and after 1 year (at the first anniversary of her surgery), she developed panic attacks. Ms. B acknowledged that the first attack had actually occurred when she was told she had cancer; however, she had been afraid to tell her psychiatrist about these symptoms. These attacks resolved with deep-breathing exercises, continued psychotherapy, and nighttime lorazepam during the anniversary crisis period. After 2 years of treatment, she was considering returning to work and starting a family.

The agoraphobic cancer patient who must be confined in an unfamiliar hospital environment and who is worried about his or her cancer may develop anxiety symptoms that need special attention. Often we make arrangements for the family of an agoraphobic patient to remain in the hospital on a 24-hour basis to provide support and reassurance during hospitalization.

Other phobias complicate the care of patients with cancer when some aspect of the diagnostic work-up and medical care leads to a confrontation with a feared situation that the patient otherwise has been able to avoid (e.g., needle phobias). Claustrophobic patients report having difficulty being moved in elevators, or being placed in scanning devices (e.g., magnetic resonance imaging and computed tomography scanners) (Brennan et al. 1988). Not infrequently, patients who have not previously reported their claustrophobia find that they cannot tolerate being confined alone in a radiation treatment room. Relaxation and distraction techniques are often helpful in decreasing anxiety, both before and during procedures. GAD is characterized by excessive, pervasive, and unrealistic anxiety that is manifested by motor tension, autonomic hyperactivity, and an increased state of alertness. In the medical setting, patients with GAD tend to anticipate complications of treatment and fear that staff will not pay sufficient attention to their symptoms.

PTSD may antedate the diagnosis of cancer or may be a result of particularly painful or frightening cancer experiences. It results from a traumatic event that is persistently reexperienced by a hypervigilant patient in a distressing manner (e.g., nightmares and intrusive thoughts). Patients either avoid stimuli that they associate with the trauma or experience a sense of emotional detachment. Symptoms often develop at the time of cancer diagnosis and can elicit feelings about earlier traumas. Individuals with a history of PTSD may experience a reemergence of their symptoms when diagnosed with cancer. We reported two such cases in a holocaust survivor and in a Vietnam War veteran (Shakin et al. 1991); however, patients who have undergone any number of traumas such as rape, accidents, or natural disasters are at risk (Madakasya and O'Brien 1987; Nadelson et al. 1982; Pitman et al. 1989).

Anxiety Related to Medical Factors

The second most frequent cause of anxiety in the cancer patient is medical factors. Medical causes of anxiety include uncontrolled pain, abnormal metabolic states, medications that produce anxiety as a side effect, withdrawal states, and, less frequently, hormone-producing tumors. DSM-III-R classifies this type of anxiety as an *organic anxiety syndrome*. Its clinical picture is similar to that of other types of anxiety.

In the cancer setting, a common factor responsible for an organic anxiety syndrome is poorly controlled acute pain. Unfortunately, undermedication of pain in oncology settings is still common. The ordering of analgesics on an as-needed basis contributes to patients' anxiety.

Suggesting that pain medications be ordered around the clock may help reduce patients' anxiety between doses (Massie and Holland 1987a).

The clinical presentation of the patient in acute pain is well known; the patient appears tense and is often restless and perspiring. If relief is not provided, agitation may develop. Suicidal ideation is common with uncontrolled pain, and psychiatric diagnoses cannot be confirmed until pain has been controlled. If anxiety persists after pain has been relieved, other medical or psychological factors should be considered, and a treatment plan can be instituted.

Symptoms of anxiety may be the first sign of a change in metabolic state or an impending catastrophic event. Suddenly occurring symptoms of anxiety with chest pain or respiratory distress may indicate a pulmonary embolus. Patients who are hypoxic from a number of causes appear anxious and are fearful that they are suffocating or dying. The bronchodilators and β-adrenergic receptor stimulants, medications that are used for chronic respiratory conditions, can cause anxiety, irritability, and tremulousness. Providing a mild sedative drug to reduce the anxiety sometimes improves breathing. The drug selected should have minimal depressant effects on the respiratory center. Low doses of the antihistamine hydroxyzine can be used for patients who have serious respiratory impairment and for those in whom physicians have other reasons to be concerned about suppression of central respiratory drive by the benzodiazepines. Short-acting benzodiazepines, such as lorazepam, are sometimes chosen in this setting.

Sepsis accompanied by chills and fever is often associated with anxiety. Delirium, irrespective of cause, may have symptoms of anxiety, restlessness, and increasing agitation. Confusional states often result from multiple causes in cancer patients: hypoglycemia, organ failure, electrolyte imbalances, nutritional failure, and/or infection (Massie et al. 1983). In patients who do not respond to the benzodiazepines or who have cognitive impairments that make them more vulnerable to benzodiazepine-related confusion and disinhibition, a neuroleptic (e.g., haloperidol) may be more useful in decreasing anxiety (Fleishman and Lesko 1989).

Among the drugs commonly used in cancer patients, the corticosteroids are frequently a cause of anxiety symptoms such as motor restlessness and agitation. Dexamethasone is often given in high doses as an emergency treatment for spinal cord compression, and prednisone often is given either as a premedication in various chemotherapy protocols to reduce nausea and vomiting or as a component of standard cancer treatment regimens. Psychiatric symptoms (e.g., anxiety symptoms, depression, and suicidal ideation) can be seen with high doses or with rapid tapering of these medications.

Akathisia is a side effect of several neuroleptic drugs (e.g., metoclopramide and prochlorperazine) that are commonly used for control of emesis in the oncology setting. It is manifested by both subjective and objective signs of restlessness. Metoclopramide is usually given intravenously as a premedication, and prochlorperazine is used orally or rectally for diminution of emetic episodes. The patient and the family are often bewildered by the "anxiety" and distress that are side effects of these medications. Fortunately, akathisia can be rapidly controlled by the addition of a benzodiazepine (e.g., lorazepam 2 mg po bid or tid), a beta-blocker (e.g., propranolol 10 mg po tid as a starting dose), or an antiparkinsonian agent (e.g., diphenhydramine 25–50 mg po or iv as a starting dose). Unfortunately, cancer patients with akathisia often fear they are now having a "nervous breakdown" and are fearful about reporting symptoms. Patients should be warned of the side effects of these antiemetic medications and encouraged to report symptoms early so treatment can be started.

Withdrawal states from alcohol, narcotic analgesics, and sedative hypnotics are often overlooked as causes of anxiety and agitation. With the trend toward shorter hospital admissions and fewer numbers of presurgical days, we are seeing an increase in delirium tremens in postsurgical patients. Patients with head and neck cancers often have histories of heavy alcohol use, and staff working with patients with head and neck cancer need to be aware that they are at increased risk for alcohol withdrawal states.

With the increasing use of the short-acting benzodiazepines (e.g., lorazepam, alprazolam, and oxazepam), we are seeing increasing amounts of rebound anxiety between doses. Patients with these symptoms often benefit from an alteration in the dose of the short-acting benzodiazepine or a switch to a longer-acting drug (e.g., diazepam and clorazepate).

Finally, hormone-secreting tumors may produce symptoms of anxiety, including panic. Pheochromocytoma, thyroid and parathyroid tumors, and adrenocorticotropic hormone (ACTH)-producing tumors (most frequently associated with lung cancer and insulinoma) are tumors that may have associated anxiety symptoms. Benzodiazepines can reduce distress while a medical workup is undertaken simultaneously and definitive treatment is planned.

Management of Anxiety in Cancer Patients

The management of anxiety is best started by a patient's primary physician who provides adequate information and support. This allows the patient to mentally "walk through" the planned surgery or treatment. Sometimes anxiety contributes to increased delays in seeking or pursuing treatment options and impairs a patient's ability to assimilate useful information from his or her physicians. This may lead to misunderstandings, to the breakdown of an adaptive patient-physician relationship, and/or to actual noncompliance. Interventions should be designed to help the patient, family members, and staff deal with the psychological issues related to or exacerbated by the cancer.

Subsequent interventions are more specific and may involve the use of multiple disciplines. They may include the use of a variety of techniques, depending on the patient's needs. Psychiatrists, psychologists, psychiatric nurse clinicians, social workers, pastoral counselors, and "veteran" cancer patients may each make important contributions to a patient's coping process. By providing support, information, and skills, these individuals can help the patient negotiate his or her way through a complex health care system. The mental health consultant can clarify the medical situation, discuss the meaning of the patient's illness, and help the patient reestablish appropriate and attainable life goals and expectations. "Veteran" patients who have survived the cancer experience can reassure the patient that "it is possible to get through all this." Group therapy and self-help groups provide additional information, reinforce positive coping strategies, and create a powerful milieu for sharing experiences. Religious counseling may provide additional support and spiritual guidance during times of emotional crisis.

Psychosocial interventions for anxiety, which can be used alone or in combination, include supportive psychotherapy, anxiolytic medications, and behavioral interventions. Brief supportive psychotherapy is often useful in dealing with crisis-related issues (Massie et al. 1989). Relaxation, guided imagery, and hypnosis may help reduce anxiety and thereby increase a patient's sense of control. In a randomized study (Holland et al. 1991) comparing a relaxation technique with alprazolam (a triazolobenzodiazepine) in the treatment of anxiety and distress in cancer patients, both treatments were demonstrated to be effective for mild to moderate degrees of anxiety or distress. The drug intervention (alprazolam) was more effective for greater levels of distress or anxiety and had more rapid onset of beneficial effect. Often, we will use such interventions in combination, that is, using relaxation techniques concurrently with anxiolytic medications in highly anxious cancer patients. Benzodiazepines can decrease daytime anxiety (e.g., lorazepam 0.5 mg po three to four times a day or alprazolam 0.25–0.5 mg po three to four times a day) or relieve insomnia (e.g., temazepam 15–30 mg or triazolam 0.125–0.250 mg po at bedtime). Buspirone (a nonbenzodiazepine anxiolytic) may be a useful adjunct in patients with chronic anxiety; however, patients who have been treated previously with benzodiazepines may find buspirone a less immediately effective treatment.

The choice of benzodiazepine depends on the desired half-life, route of administration available, route of metabolism, and the presence or absence of active metabolites (Table 1–3). In the medically ill

Table 1–3.   Commonly prescribed benzodiazepines in cancer patients

Drug name (by class)	Approximate dose equivalent	Initial dosage (mg po)	Elimination half-life drug metabolites (hours)	Active metabolite
Short acting				
Alprazolam	0.5	0.25–0.5 tid	10–15	Yes
Oxazepam	10.0	10–15 tid	5–15	No
Lorazepam[a]	1.0	0.5–2.0 tid	10–20	No
Temazepam[b]	15.0	15–30 qhs	10–15	No
Triazolam[b]	0.25	0.125–0.25 qhs	1–5	No
Intermediate acting				
Chlordiazepoxide	10.0	10–25 tid	10–40	Yes
Long acting				
Diazepam	5.0	5–10 bid	20–100	Yes
Clorazepate	7.5	7.5–15 bid	30–200	Yes

Note.   tid = three times a day; bid = twice a day; qhs = at bedtime.
[a]Lorazepam can also be administered parenterally; other benzodiazepines are erratically absorbed when given parenterally.
[b]Hypnotic agent.

patient, drugs with shorter half-lives, multiple routes of administration, and no active metabolites are preferable. In patients with hepatic disease the benzodiazepines of choice are the short-acting compounds (e.g., oxazepam and lorazepam) that are metabolized primarily by conjugation and are excreted by the kidney. Cancer patients frequently need to be encouraged to take sufficient amounts of medication to provide relief from anxiety. The persistence of side effects, such as drowsiness, motor incoordination, and confusion, necessitates dose reduction or discontinuation. Behavioral disinhibition is rarely noted.

Benzodiazepines are usually readily discontinued by cancer patients when the symptoms of anxiety abate but should be tapered slowly to avoid symptoms of withdrawal. Concerns about addiction should not interfere with their use in the cancer setting (Massie and Lesko 1989).

To control anxiety before chemotherapy or painful procedures, the short-acting benzodiazepine lorazepam is useful because it provides anterograde amnesia, both after oral and intravenous administration. Lorazepam is also rapidly absorbed via the sublingual route. Lorazepam reduces vomiting when given intravenously with other antiemetics and reduces vomiting in patients receiving highly emetic chemotherapy regimens (e.g., cisplatin). Lorazepam alone often does not decrease the number or frequency of emetic events; however, patients remember little of their vomiting episodes (Bishop et al. 1984; Laszlo et al. 1985). Alprazolam given for 1–2 days and then just before chemotherapy has been demonstrated to reduce anticipatory nausea and vomiting in cancer patients (Greenberg et al. 1987)

Although acute and chronic anxiety states in cancer patients are usually treated with benzodiazepines, antipsychotic medications in low doses (e.g., thioridazine 10 mg tid) can be used with severe anxiety when an adequate dose of a benzodiazepine is not effective. Antihistamines are generally less effective as anxiolytics (Jenike 1983).

Summary

The management of anxiety and depression in cancer patients requires a multidisciplinary and multimodal approach. The combined use of psychotherapy, behavioral techniques, and the somatic therapies has proven to be an effective means of helping patients negotiate their way through the extremely stressful process of the diagnosis and treatment of cancer.

References

American Psychiatric Association: Diagnostic and Statistical Manual of Mental Disorders, 3rd Edition. Washington, DC, American Psychiatric Association, 1980

American Psychiatric Association: Diagnostic and Statistical Manual of Mental Disorders, 3rd Edition, Revised. Washington, DC, American Psychiatric Association, 1987

Bishop JF, Oliver IN, Wolf MM, et al: Lorazepam: a randomized, double-blind, cross-over study of a new antiemetic in patients receiving cytotoxic chemotherapy and prochlorperazine. J Clin Oncol 2:691–695, 1984

Breitbart W: Suicide in cancer patients. Oncology 1:49–53, 1987

Breitbart W: Suicide in cancer patients, in Handbook of Psychooncology: Psychological Care of the Patient With Cancer. Edited by Holland JC, Rowland JH. New York, Oxford University Press, 1989, pp 291–299

Breitbart W, Holland JC: Psychiatric complications of cancer. Current Therapy in Hematology-Oncology 3:268–274, 1988

Brennan SC, Redd WH, Jacobsen PB, et al: Anxiety and panic during magnetic resonance scans (letter). Lancet 2:512, 1988

Bruera E, Breuneis C, Paterson AH, et al: Use of methylphenidate as an adjuvant to narcotic analgesics in patients with advanced cancer. Journal of Pain and Symptom Management 4:3–6, 1989

Bukberg JB, Penman DT, Holland JC: Depression in hospitalized cancer patients. Psychosom Med 46:199–212, 1984

Cancer chemotherapy. Med Lett Drugs Ther 29:29–36, 1987

Chiarello RJ, Cole JO: The use of psychostimulants in general psychiatry: a reconsideration. Arch Gen Psychiatry 44:286–295, 1987

Cooper GL: The safety of fluoxetine: an update. Br J Psychiatry 153(suppl 3):77–86, 1988

Derogatis LR, Morrow GR, Fetting J, et al: The prevalence of psychiatric disorders among cancer patients. JAMA 249:751–757, 1983

Drugs of choice for cancer chemotherapy. Med Lett Drugs Ther 33:21–28, 1991

Drugs that cause psychiatric symptoms. Med Lett Drugs Ther 31:113–118, 1989

Fernandez F, Adams F, Holmes VF, et al: Methylphenidate for depressive disorders in cancer patients. Psychosomatics 28:455–461, 1987

Fleishman SB, Lesko LM: Delirium and dementia, in Handbook of Psychooncology: Psychological Care of the Patient With Cancer. Edited by Holland JC, Rowland JH. New York, Oxford University Press, 1989, pp 342–355

France RD: The future for antidepressants: treatment of pain. Psychopathology 20:99–113, 1987

Glassman AH: The newer antidepressant drugs and their cardiovascular effects. Psychopharmacol Bull 20:272–279, 1984

Greenberg DB, Surman OS, Clarke J, et al: Alprazolam or phobic nausea and vomiting related to chemotherapy. Cancer Treatment Reports 71:549–550, 1987

Hinton J: Psychiatric consultation in fatal illness. Proc R Soc Med 65:29–32, 1972

Holland JC, Hughes-Korzun A, Tross S, et al: Comparative psychological disturbance in pancreatic and gastric cancer. Am J Psychiatry 143:982–986, 1986

Holland JC, Rowland JH, Lebovits A, et al: Reactions to cancer treatment: assessment of emotional response to adjuvant radiotherapy as a guide to planned interventions. Psychiatr Clin North Am 2:347–358, 1979

Holland JC, Morrow G, Schmale A, et al: A randomized clinical trial of alprazolam versus progressive muscle relaxation in cancer patients with anxiety and depressive symptoms. J Clin Oncol 9:1004–1011, 1991

Jenike MA: Treating anxiety in elderly patients. Geriatrics 38:115–119, 1983

Koenig R, Levin SM, Brennan MJ: The emotional status of cancer patients as measured by a psychological test. Journal of Chronic Disease 20:923–930, 1967

Lansky SB, List MA, Herrmann CA, et al: Absence of major depressive disorder in female cancer patients. J Clin Oncol 3:1553–1560, 1985

Laszlo J, Clark RA, Hanson DC, et al: Lorazepam in cancer patients treated with cisplatin: a drug having antiemetic, amnesic and anxiolytic effects. J Clin Oncol 3:864–869, 1985

Locke BZ, Reiger DA: Prevalence of selected mental disorders, in Mental Health United States. Edited by Janke CA, Barrell SA. Rockville, MD, National Institute of Mental Health, 1985, pp 1–6

Madakasya S, O'Brien KF: Acute post traumatic stress disorder in victims of a natural disaster. J Nerv Ment Dis 175:286–290, 1987

Massie MJ: Anxiety, panic, and phobias, in Handbook of Psychooncology: Psychological Care of the Patient With Cancer. Edited by Holland JC, Rowland JH. New York, Oxford University Press, 1989a, pp 300–309

Massie MJ: Depression, in Handbook of Psychooncology: Psychological Care of the Patient With Cancer. Edited by Holland JC, Rowland JH. New York, Oxford University Press, 1989b, pp 283–290

Massie MJ, Holland JC: Consultation and liaison issues in cancer care. Psychiatr Med 5:343–359, 1987a

Massie MJ, Holland JC: The cancer patient with pain: psychiatric complications and their management. Med Clin North Am 71:243–258, 1987b

Massie MJ, Holland JC: Overview of normal reactions and prevalence of psychiatric disorders, in Handbook of Psychooncology: Psychological Care of the Patient With Cancer. Edited by Holland JC, Rowland JH. New York, Oxford University Press, 1989, pp 273–282

Massie MJ, Lesko L: Psychopharmacological management, in Handbook of Psychooncology: Psychological Care of the Patient With Cancer. Edited by Holland JC, Rowland JH. New York, Oxford University Press, 1989, pp 470–491

Massie MJ, Holland JC, Glass E: Delirium in terminally ill cancer patients. Am J Psychiatry 140:1048–1050, 1983

Massie MJ, Holland JC, Straker N: Psychotherapeutic interventions, in Handbook of Psychooncology: Psychological Care of the Patient With Cancer. Edited by Holland JC, Rowland JH. New York, Oxford University Press, 1989, pp 455–469

Moffic H, Paykel ES: Depression in medical inpatients. Br J Psychiatry 126:346–353, 1975

Nadelson CC, Notman MT, Zackson H, et al: A follow-up study of rape victims. Am J Psychiatry 139:1266–1270, 1982

Pitman RK, Altman B, Macklin MI: Prevalence of post traumatic stress disorder in wounded Vietnam veterans. Am J Psychiatry 146:667–669, 1989

Plumb M, Holland JC: Comparative studies of psychological function in patients with advanced cancer, I: self-reported depressive symptoms. Psychosom Med 39:264–276, 1977

Schwab JJ, Bialon M, Brown JM, et al: Diagnosing depression in medical inpatients. Ann Intern Med 67:695–707, 1967

Scott DW: Anxiety: critical thinking and information processing during and after breast biopsy. Nurs Res 32:24–28, 1983

Shakin EJ, Holland JC: Depression and pancreatic cancer. Journal of Pain and Symptom Management 3:194–198, 1988

Shakin EJ, Heiligenstein E, Holland J: Psychiatric complications of cancer, in The Complications of Cancer Management. Edited by Plowman PN, McElwain TJ, Meadows AT. Guilford, England, Butterworth Scientific, 1991, pp 423–435

Stiefel FC, Breitbart WS, Holland JC: Corticosteroids in cancer: neuropsychiatric complications. Cancer Invest 7:479–491, 1989

Chapter 2

Treatment of Organic Mental Disorders in Cancer Patients

Stewart B. Fleishman, M.D.
Lynna M. Lesko, M.D., Ph.D.
William Breitbart, M.D.

*O*rganic mental disorders are unfortunately all too common in patients with cancer. Delirium, dementia, organic mood and anxiety, or organic personality disorders can result from either direct or indirect effects of cancer or its treatment on the central nervous system (CNS). Psychiatric symptoms and behavioral changes resulting from organic mental disorders, particularly in milder early stages, are often mistakenly attributed to the emotional impact of cancer or possible depression. Psychiatrists working in the cancer setting must not only provide support for patients, family, and staff, they must also function as psychiatric physicians providing diagnostic and treatment services for patients with such CNS complications of cancer. Early recognition of acute organic mental disorders is critical to both treatment efficacy and prevention of progression to more severe organic states or chronic, treatment-resistant forms such as dementia. Psychiatrists play a vital role in the accurate diagnosis and proper treatment of such disorders in cancer patients. In this chapter, we review the issues related to diagnostic criteria, prevalence, etiology, and management of organic mental disorders in the oncology setting.

Diagnostic Criteria of Organic Mental Disorders in Cancer Patients

DSM-III-R (American Psychiatric Association 1987) divides organic mental syndromes into the subcategories of delirium, dementia, amnestic syndrome, organic hallucinosis, organic delusional syndrome, organic mood syndrome, organic anxiety syndrome, organic personality syndrome, intoxications, and withdrawal states. Although virtually all of these organic mental syndromes can be seen in cancer patients, the most common include delirium, dementia, organic mood syndrome, and organic anxiety syndrome.

Lipowski (1987) categorized organic mental disorders into those that were characterized by general cognitive impairment (i.e., delirium and dementia) and those in which cognitive impairment was rather selective or limited (i.e., amnestic disorder, organic hallucinosis, and so on). The DSM-III-R classification provides a set of explicit diagnostic criteria for differentiating the various organic mental syndromes and disorders (a distinction is made between organic mental *syndromes* and organic mental *disorders*). *Organic mental disorder* describes an organic mental syndrome in which an etiology is known or presumed, as in the case of an organic delusional disorder due to a brain malignancy (American Psychiatric Association 1987). In this chapter, we use DSM-III-R terminology wherever possible and practical. For simplicity, however, the term *organic mental disorders* is used to refer generically to the entire spectrum of organic mental syndromes and disorders.

Delirium has been characterized as an etiologically nonspecific organic cerebral dysfunction characterized by concurrent disturbances of level of consciousness, attention, thinking, perception, memory, psychomotor behavior, emotion, and the sleep-wake cycle. Disorientation and fluctuation, or waxing and waning of the above symptoms, as well as an abrupt temporal onset of such disturbances, are other important features of delirium.

At times it is difficult to differentiate delirium from dementia because they frequently share common clinical features such as impaired memory, thinking, and judgment and disorientation (Table 2–1). Liston (1984) outlined the major diagnostic differences between the clinical pictures of delirium and dementia. Dementia appears in relatively alert individuals with little or no clouding of consciousness. The temporal onset of symptoms in dementia is more subacute or chronically progressive, and the sleep-wake cycle of individuals with dementia seems less impaired. Most prominent in dementia are difficulties in short- and long-term memory and impaired judgment and abstract thinking, as well as disturbed higher cortical functions (e.g., aphasia and apraxia). Occasionally elderly patients will have a delirium super-imposed on an underlying dementia.

Other types of organic mental disorders are characterized by rela-tively intact cognition, but with 1) more selective impairment as in amnestic syndrome or disorder or 2) more prominent symptoms con-sisting of anxiety, mood disturbance, delusions, hallucinations, or per-sonality change. For instance, patients with mood disturbance meeting criteria for major depression, who are severely hypothyroid or on high-dose corticosteroids are most accurately diagnosed as having an organic mood disorder, depressed type (particularly if the organic factors are judged to be the primary etiology related to the disturbance). Similarly, patients with hyponatremia or patients on acyclovir for CNS herpes, who are experiencing visual hallucinations but have an intact sensorium with minimal cognitive deficits, are more accurately diag-nosed as having an organic hallucinosis.

Proposed changes for DSM-IV call for the category of organic mental disorders to be eliminated on the grounds that the label *organic*

Table 2–1.   Clinical features of delirium and dementia

Feature	Delirium	Dementia
Impaired memory	+++	+++
Impaired thinking	+++	+++
Impaired judgment	+++	+++
Clouding of consciousness	+++	—
Major attention deficits	+++	+
Fluctuation over course of day	+++	+
Disorientation	+++	++
Vivid perceptual disturbances	++	+
Incoherent speech	++	+
Disrupted sleep-wake cycle	++	+
Nocturnal exacerbation	++	+
Insight	++	+
Acute or subacute onset	++	—

Note.   +++ = Always present; ++ = usually present; + = present sometime; — = usually absent.
Source.   Adapted from Liston EH: "Diagnosis and Management of Delirium in the Elderly." *Psychiatric Annals* 14:109–118, 1984.

has lost its specificity in the era of biological psychiatry (in which a wide variety of traditionally functional or "nonorganic" mental disorders have now been demonstrated to have biological and neurophysiological etiologies). The DSM-IV organic disorders work group is proposing that the "traditional" organic mental disorders (i.e., dementia, delirium, and amnestic syndrome or disorder) be recategorized as "cognitive disorders" and that the remaining organic mental disorders (i.e., organic mood syndrome or disorder, organic anxiety syndrome or disorder, organic hallucinosis, organic delusional syndrome or disorder, and organic personality syndrome or disorder) be included within the diagnostic categories that share phenomenology (Lipowski 1990; Tucker et al. 1990). For example, under these proposed changes organic mood syndrome or disorder would be classified with the affective disorders, organic delusional syndrome or disorder would be classified with the psychotic disorders, and both would be referred to as "symptomatic" or secondary disorders.

Prevalence of Organic Mental Disorders

Estimates of the prevalence of delirium in cancer patients range from 8% to 40% (Derogatis et al. 1983; Levine et al. 1978). This variability is explained by differences in type of cancer, the setting in which patients are treated, and whether patient data are collected in a random fashion from various hospital floors or psychiatric consultation data are used. In addition, the screening technique (e.g., clinical psychiatric interview, semistructured interview, and neuropsychological inventory) affects prevalence rates.

There are three groups of cancer patients at risk for increased incidence of delirium: patients who are under treatment in the hospital, those who are older (Seymour et al. 1980), and those who have more advanced or terminal disease (Massie et al. 1983). Hospitalized patients in general are at increased risk of developing a narcotic- or steroid-induced confusional state or a metabolic encephalopathy related to the consequences of disease or treatment. Posner (1979) estimated that 15% to 20% of patients on medical oncology units may be experiencing some degree of cognitive impairment, usually not recognized unless severe or accompanied by behavioral changes.

The prevalence of dementia in the cancer setting, usually from unusual remote effects on the CNS or from radiation, is low. DeAngelis et al. (1989) reviewed 370 cases and reported on 12 cases (3%) of radiation-induced dementia in patients cured of their brain metastases. Within a range of 5–36 months these patients developed a severe and progressive dementia accompanied by ataxia and urinary incontinence. This syndrome appeared similar to a subcortical dementia and was fatal in 7 out of the 12 patients.

Etiology of Organic Mental Disorders

The causes of organic mental disorders in cancer patients are outlined in Table 2–2. Posner (1978, 1988) outlined two main etiologies of CNS complications: 1) direct effects related to primary brain tumors or metastatic spread by local extension or by hematogenous or lymphatic routes, which may result in delirium or permanent intellectual loss or dementia, and 2) indirect effects, which are far more frequent and more commonly cause delirium, such as organ failure, electrolyte imbalance, endocrine abnormalities, drug or radiation side effects, infection, vascular complications, nutritional changes, and paraneoplastic syndromes.

Table 2–2.   Causes of organic mental disorders in cancer patients

Direct
    Primary brain tumor
    Metastatic spread

Indirect
    Metabolic encephalopathy due to organ failure
    Electrolyte imbalance
    Treatment side effects from
        Chemotherapeutic agents, steroids, and biological response
            modifiers
        Radiation
        Narcotics
        Anticholinergics
        Antiemetics
    Infection
    Hematologic abnormalities
    Nutrition
    Paraneoplastic syndromes

Direct Causes

Patchell and Posner (1989) provided an excellent review on organic mental disorders caused by direct invasion of the CNS by primary brain tumors or metastatic disease. Primary brain tumors account for approximately 3% of cancer deaths and have an incidence of about 10 per 100,000 people (Patchell and Posner 1989). They are unfortunately the second most common type of tumor diagnosed in children. The neurological symptoms of such primary CNS tumors depend on each tumor's location and involvement. Posterior fossa tumors cause increased intracranial pressure resulting in headache, nausea, vomiting, gait abnormalities, and lethargy, whereas hemispheric tumors cause seizures, headache, visual field deficits, weakness, aphasia, sensory disturbances, and dementia, rather than delirium. Metastatic spread of a tumor (e.g., melanoma, lung, colon, breast, and renal cell) to the brain is quite common, with 25% of patients who die having an intracranial lesion at the time of their death. These lesions can appear anywhere in the brain but usually predominate in the "watershed" areas of the cerebral hemisphere, spread by hematogenous routes. Presenting symptoms and complaints by patients usually consist of headache followed by numerous focal neurological deficits or seizures (in 15% of patients); approximately 1% to 2% of patients have a "nonfocal encephalopathy" (Patchell and Posner 1989). Treatment of neuropsychiatric complications of primary or metastatic invasion of the CNS often involves both behavioral and pharmacological interventions.

Indirect Causes

Metabolic and endocrine disorders. Metabolic and endocrine abnormalities are common in the cancer setting and are frequent causes of organic mental disorders (Table 2–3). Failure of a vital organ (particularly liver, kidney, lung, thyroid, or adrenal gland) is a common source of mental status change in patients with advanced disease, elderly patients, and patients with other medical illnesses complicating their cancer course. Uremia and hepatic dysfunction can produce an encephalopathy with neuropsychiatric symptoms ranging from mild lethargy to coma. Respiratory compromise from tumor extension, chemotherapy-induced fibrosis, or preexisting pulmonary disease can of course produce hypoxia and resulting confusion. Hyponatremia or

Table 2–3. Organic mental disorders seen with metabolic and endocrine abnormalities in cancer patients

Abnormality	Organic mood disorder		Delirium	Dementia	Organic delusional disorder	Organic anxiety disorder	Organic personality disorder
	Depressed	Manic					
Hypercortisolism	+++	++	++	+	+++	+	+
Hypocortisolism	++	−	+	+	+	−	+
Hyperthyroidism	+	+	++	+	++	+++	+
Hypothyroidism	+++	−	++	+	++	−	−
Hypercalcemia	++	−	++	++	++	−	+
Hypocalcemia	+	+	+++	++	+	+++	−
Hyperglycemia	−	−	+	++	−	−	−
Hypoglycemia	++	+	+++	++	++	+++	+
Hyponatremia (SIADH)	++	−	++	++	+	−	−
Hypokalemia	++	−	++	++	+	+	−
Hypophosphatemia	+	−	++	+	−	++	++
Carcinoid	+	−	+	−	−	−	−
Pheochromocytoma	−	−	−	−	−	+++	++

Note. +++ = frequent; ++ = common; + = rare; SIADH = sustained inappropriate antidiuretic hormone.
Source. Adapted from Breitbart WB: "Endocrine-Related Psychiatric Disorders," in *Handbook of Psychooncology: Psychological Care of the Patient With Cancer.* Edited by Holland JC, Rowland JH. New York, Oxford University Press, 1989, pp. 356–366.

hypokalemia from vomiting, diarrhea, or hyperalimentation can cause lethargy and weakness accompanied by perceptual cognitive or memory changes. Endocrine disorders of cortisol, thyroid, calcium, glucose, and sodium metabolic regulation can all contribute to neuropsychiatric symptomatology in cancer patients (Table 2–3). (For a comprehensive review, see Breitbart 1989.)

Steroid-producing tumors of the adrenal gland, tumors of the hypothalamic-pituitary axis, ectopic adrenocorticotropic hormone production (from lung, pancreas, thyroid, and pheocromocytoma), and exogenous administration of steroid medication can all produce a syndrome of hypercortisolism and subsequent psychiatric manifestations (Haskett 1985). Many of the above conditions are rare and only a portion of them produce enough cortisol to produce Cushing's syndrome. However, it is noteworthy that exogenously administered corticosteroids are routinely used in cancer treatment protocols and are the most common cause of hypercortisolism. Mild affective (e.g., irritability and anxiety) and cognitive (e.g., impaired memory and concentration) disturbances are common with hypercortisolism. Major psychiatric disturbances such as mania, depression, delirium, or reversible dementia can develop in a small but unpredictable population of patients (Stiefel et al. 1989). Higher doses of steroid appear to be correlated with increased risk of psychiatric symptoms, but neuropsychiatric disturbance can occur at any dose range (Boston Collaborative Drug Surveillance Program 1972).

Thyroid cancer is extremely rare with a prevalence of less than 1%. Hyperthyroidism secondary to a hyperfunctional thyroid nodule is equally as rare. Psychiatric symptomatology from hyperthyroidism, if present, typically presents with anxiety, affective complaints, cognitive impairment, and even psychosis (Taylor 1973). Hypothyroidism in the cancer setting, due to surgery or ablative ^{131}I radiotherapy, can cause a subcortical dementia (difficulty in concentrating, short-term memory loss, and psychomotor slowing), depression, and rarely "myxedema madness" (an organic affective disorder with delirium) (Touks 1974).

Hypercalcemia, common in multiple myeloma, lung cancer, ovarian cancer, and, less often, prostate cancer, can occur as a result of bone invasion via metastases or of the effects on bone by several humoral mediators resembling osteoclast-activating factor, parathyroid hormone, and growth hormone (Mundy and Martin 1982). Calcium levels between 12 and 16 mg/dl are associated with primarily affective disturbances (e.g., apathy, slowed cognition, and depression); levels between 16 and 19 mg/dl are usually associated with symptoms of delirium (e.g., confusion, disorientation, hallucinations, and paranoia). Levels greater than 20 mg/dl usually result in somnolence and coma (Smith et al. 1972).

Very high levels of serum glucose are not usually a problem in the cancer setting. Several chemotherapy agents such as L-asparaginase, vincristine, and streptozocin can interfere with glucose regulation and cause hyperglycemia (Breitbart 1989). It should be remembered, however, that hyperosmolar states produced by very high serum glucose levels can result in an encephalopathy, producing coma and death. Hypoglycemia can develop from rare insulinomas, mesenchymal tumors, and hepatomas. Abrupt changes in serum glucose levels can result in pallor, tachycardia, anxiety (glucose levels less than 70 mg/dl), myoclonic twitching, seizures, and frank delirium (glucose levels less than 40 mg/dl) (Sachs 1973).

Forty percent of patients with oat-cell carcinoma of the lung develop ectopic secretion of antidiuretic hormone (ADH) resulting in sustained inappropriate antidiuretic hormone (SIADH) syndrome (Gilbey et al. 1975). This syndrome, which is characterized by hyponatremia, renal sodium loss, and hypervolemia, can also be seen with prostate cancer, Hodgkin's disease, and the use of chemotherapy agents such as vincristine and cyclophosphamide. Serum sodium levels that drop to less than 120 mg/dl are associated with confusion, cognitive impairment, delirium, and seizures (Sandifer 1983). Hypophosphatemia and hypomagnesemia (Schilsky and Anderson 1979) can result from treatment with cisplatin (a common chemotherapeutic agent) and may cause weakness, delirium, irritability, apprehension, and even somnolence, coma, and death. The following case example illustrates how there may be a significant lag from the time or normalization of a metabolic disturbance to the time of resolution of psychiatric symptoms:

Case 1

Mr. C, a usually quiet and pleasant 68-year-old man, had been admitted to the hospital after a 36-hour period of nausea, vomiting, and weakness 4 days after receiving cisplatin as part of a chemotherapy protocol for lung cancer. He was afebrile without sepsis. On admission blood work, Mr. C's inorganic phosphorous was noted to be 1.4 mg/dl (normal range 3.0–4.5 mg/dl). Despite slow replacement of phosphates intravenously, he became progressively weaker and developed areflexia, decreased sensation in the lower extremities, cranial nerve weakness, and extensor plantar reflexes. Because he was unable to eat at all, hyperalimentation was begun. He became more tired but irascible, showing little tolerance for usual nursing routines like blood drawing. Within 5 days of the return of his phosphorus level to a normal range he was able to tolerate liquids and then solid food, and hyperalimentation was discontinued. He became more compliant with the demands of hospital care and felt stronger. Objectively, the generalized and cranial nerve weakness reversed. Mr. C was discharged to await the next cycle of his chemotherapy.

Infections of the CNS produce an encephalopathy secondary to bacterial, viral, or fungal invasion of the brain. Some of the nutritional deficiencies seen in cancer and associated with mental status changes are thiamine deficiency, which produces Wernicke-Korsakoff syndrome, and folic acid and vitamin B12 deficiency, which can also produce progressive cognitive impairment and dementia. Patients with carcinoid syndrome can develop a niacin deficiency secondary to tryptophan "steal" syndrome. Pellagra can result with the triad of dermatitis, diarrhea, and dementia (Major et al. 1973; Patchell and Posner 1986).

Chemotherapy. Many antineoplastic agents cross the blood-brain barrier in sufficient quantities to directly cause cognitive, memory, and perceptual changes, even delirium (Fleishman and Lesko 1989; Kaplan and Wiernik 1983; Young and Posner 1980). Table 2–4 presents a complete list of the CNS symptoms and toxicity of the classic cytotoxic agents as well as the newer biological modifiers. Of the classic chemotherapeutic agents, methotrexate, 5-fluororacil, the vinca alkaloids, bleomycins, cisplatin, L-asparaginase, and procarbazine are the most commonly associated with the production of neuropsychiatric disturbances, especially delirium (Young and Posner 1980).

High-dose regimens of methotrexate or cytosine arabinoside can also cause a leukoencephalopathy and a progressive dementia. Methotrexate can cause a delirium, most likely due to direct neurotoxic effects, by altering the blood-brain barrier and reducing glucose phosphorylation in the brain (Kaplan and Wiernik 1983). Positron-emission

Table 2–4. Central nervous system symptoms and toxicity of major chemotherapeutic agents used for cancer

Agent	Del	Let	Hal	Dem	Dep	Per	Man	Psy	EPS	Cog	Cer
Aminoglutethimide										X	
L-Asparaginase	X	X	X							X	
5-Azacytidine										X	
Bleomycin	X										
Carmustine (BCNU)	X			X							
Cisplatin	X										
Cytosine arabinoside (ara-C)	X	X								X	X
Dacarbazine				X							
Fludarabine	X			X						X	
Fluorouracil	X								X		
Hexylmethylamine			X								
Hydroxyurea			X								
Imidazolecarboxaminde (DITC)										X	
Interferon	X	X	X		X						
Interleukin	X	X	X					X		X	
Isophosphamide	X	X	X								
Methotrexate	X	X		X		X					
Prednisone	X		X		X	X	X	X		X	
Procarbazine	X	X	X		X		X				
Vinblastine	X	X	X		X		X				
Vincristine	X	X	X		X						

Note. Del = delirium; Let = lethargy; Hal = hallucination; Dem = dementia; Dep = depression; Per = "personality change"; Man = mania; Psy = psychosis; EPS = extra pyramidal symptoms; Cog = cognitive dysfunction; Cer = cerebellar dysfunction.

tomography (PET) scanning can help differentiate delirium caused by methotrexate from the dementia of chronic leukoencephalopathy. There is marked depression of cerebral glucose metabolism seen with methotrexate-induced delirium (Phillips et al. 1987). Approximately 50% of patients develop signs of meningeal irritation or confusion hours after intrathecal methotrexate administration (Kaplan and Wiernik 1983).

Vincristine and the other vinca alkaloids can cause delirium as well as other neurotoxicities. Vincristine neurotoxicity is usually related to the age of the patient and the dose of drug, with delirium being reported with high dosage (Legha 1986). Procarbazine can cause lethargy and confusion, or delirium, in up to 10% of patients (Kaplan and Wiernik 1983). Procarbazine is a monoamine oxidase inhibitor (MAOI) that can interact adversely with other MAOIs or narcotic analgesics such as meperidine, causing delirium, hypertension, hyperpyrexia, and cardiovascular collapse.

Encephalopathy or delirium has been reported in as many as 20% to 60% of patients treated with L-asparaginase (Holland et al. 1974; Kaplan and Wiernik 1983). Cerebrovascular complications, such as hemorrhage or thrombosis, are not uncommon with this agent (Feinberg and Swenson 1988). L-Asparaginase-induced delirium is usually reversible, but more chronic forms of confusional states have been reported. Cisplatin can cause a delirium, often as a result of magnesium depletion (Matzen and Martin 1985). Hexamethymelamine can cause delirium with hallucinations and mood disturbance (Kaplan and Wiernik 1983). Chemotherapy drugs can also cause organic mental disorders through indirect effects on the CNS, such as the production of metabolic derangements or organ failure. Vincristine may cause excessive release of antidiuretic hormone resulting in hyponatremia and delirium (Legha 1986). Doxorubicin (Adriamycin)-related cardiomyopathy can lead to congestive heart failure. Cisplatin is known to be nephrotoxic, and bleomycin-induced pulmonary fibrosis can lead to hypoxia (Silberfarb and Oxman 1988).

Corticosteroids are widely used in cancer treatment. Glucocorticoids, such as hydrocortisone, are often part of standard protocols for leukemia or lymphoma. Dexamethasone is often used as an antiemetic, an adjuvant analgesic, and to relieve CNS edema with cord compression or brain metastases. Initially, many patients experience a sense of well-being and even gain weight on corticosteroids. However, adverse neuropsychiatric complications may affect as many as 57% of patients on steroids. Adverse psychiatric symptoms range from minor mood and sleep disturbances to major affective and cognitive disorders. Euphoria is reported in as many as 30% of patients, but major psychiatric disorders occur in perhaps 5% to 10%.

Affective disorders (e.g., depression or mania) and psychotic reactions (e.g, delirium or steroid psychosis) are the most common of the clinically significant disturbances encountered (Stiefel et al. 1989). Steroid psychosis is often characterized by global cognitive impairment, which is often associated with hallucinations or delusions of a paranoid or religious nature (Hall et al. 1979). These disorders are more likely to occur with higher doses of steroids, and symptoms can persist for several days to weeks after discontinuation of steroids. The following case example illustrates commonly encountered corticosteroid-induced psychiatric symptoms:

Case 2

Ms. D, a 40-year-old woman, was diagnosed as having metastatic lung cancer after developing diplopia while driving. She was given whole-brain radiation and dexamethasone 4 mg qid, resulting in complete resolution of the focal neurological symptoms. There were no cognitive or memory deficits resulting from either illness or treatment. Apart from refraining from driving, Ms. D returned to her usual functional capacity.

Soon after the dexamethasone was begun, Ms. D felt unusually optimistic about her situation. Her appetite increased dramatically and she gained 42 lb. She had trouble both falling and staying asleep. Her family and co-workers noted that she was loud, irritable, and had a "short fuse" unlike anyone could remember. She could not concentrate enough to learn a new computer system at work. Initially, Ms. D was calmer and better able to sleep when alprazolam 0.5 mg tid and triazolam 0.25 mg at bedtime were added to her regimen, but she subjectively felt best and seemed "more like herself" to family members when haloperidol 0.5 mg and 1 mg at bedtime was substituted.

Immunotherapy. Adoptive immunotherapy and the use of biological modifiers represent promising new developments in cancer treatment. Neuropsychiatric disturbances have been reported with several immune agents including interferon (Adams et al. 1984; Quesada et al. 1986) and interleukin-2 (Denicoff et al. 1987). Adoptive immunotherapy with interleukin-2 and lymphokine-activated killer (LAK) cells can be complicated by cognitive impairment, disorientation, confusion, and mental slowing, as well as by visual hallucinations, particularly when administered in high doses. These neuropsychiatric toxicities can be treatment limiting and often appear several days after treatment has begun. This marked latency period is characterized by more subtle premonitory changes that include irritability and decreased attention and concentration (Denicoff et al. 1987).

Interferon-α can cause fatigue, a flu-like syndrome with fever, chills, a general sense of malaise, headache, nausea, and vomiting. It can also cause a change in the level of consciousness, disorientation, psychotic thinking, and hallucinations (Adams et al. 1984). An organic mood (depressive) disorder that seems to be dose related is also associated with its use. Fever, fatigue, rigors, hypotension, and cognitive and memory impairments have been reported with both interleukin-2 and tumor necrosis factor.

Radiation therapy. Whole-brain radiation, used to treat primary as well as metastatic lesions of the brain, can be complicated by a radiation-induced encephalopathy. Three types of encephalopathic syndromes have been described: 1) acute encephalopathy (seen immediately after first radiation treatment), 2) early delayed encephalopathy (beginning 6–16 weeks after treatment), and 3) late delayed encephalopathy (seen 6 months to several years later) (Patchell and Posner 1989; Sheline 1980).

Acute encephalopathy can occur during the immediate course of high-dose radiation therapy. Patients can become lethargic and complain of headache, nausea and vomiting, and fever. It is thought that this type of acute reaction is caused by increased intracranial pressure secondary to radiation-induced changes in the blood-brain barrier. Left untreated it can lead to worsening of neurological deficits and even brain herniation. Corticosteroids, particularly dexamethasone, are the treatment of choice for this syndrome.

An early delayed encephalopathy can begin 1–4 months after radiation treatment but has been reported earlier or later. Symptoms consist of lethargy, headache, nausea, and vomiting. In children who receive whole-brain radiation therapy prophylactically for leukemia, the picture is usually one of generalized somnolence and headache.

Patients who receive more focal radiation therapy to the brain can present with symptoms of focal neurological disease suggestive of recurrence of tumor. The cause of early delayed radiation encephalopathy is unknown, but it may be related to radiation-induced edema or demyelination. Improvement in symptoms usually occurs spontaneously in 1–6 weeks. Steroids may be helpful in treating symptoms as well as for prophylaxis before radiation therapy.

A late delayed encephalopathy (usually severe and permanent) may develop 6 months to 3 years (average 12 months) after radiation therapy. This syndrome is characterized by symptoms that suggest a focal neurological lesion, accompanied by personality change and headache. Seizures can also complicate the picture. Differential diagnosis includes recurrent tumor, infarct, and abscess. Computed tomography (CT) scan of the brain usually reveals a hypodense lesion in the white matter. Biopsy of brain shows necrosis. Steroids can help symptomatically; however, surgical resection of the necrotic mass is often necessary.

Paraneoplastic syndromes. "Remote effects" of cancer on the nervous system are quite rare. These paraneoplastic syndromes include a number of neurological complications of systemic cancer that are not caused by direct tumor invasion or metastases of the nervous system. Rather, their cause is unknown, although an autoimmune etiology is speculated (Patchell and Posner 1989). Paraneoplastic syndromes affecting the brain and nervous system occur in fewer than 1% of cancer patients, but are included here because of their potential to present as psychiatric disturbances, particularly organic mental disorders such as dementia and organic mood disorder (depressed). Table 2–5 lists the paraneoplastic syndromes that affect the brain, spinal cord, and neuromuscular system. These syndromes are separated into anatomical categories for the purposes of description, but there is considerable overlap of clinical presentation. For example, limbic encephalitis, cerebellar degeneration, and bulbar or brain stem encephalitis can all present with dementia.

Limbic encephalitis (Caincross 1989) can present with dementia, memory loss, mood change, and hallucinations or delusions. This paraneoplastic syndrome is a rare neurological complication of lung and other cancers. The characteristic symptoms of dementia and memory loss can however be caused by other complications of cancer such as cerebral metastases, meningeal carcinomatosis, CNS infection, or metabolic derangements. Limbic encephalitis therefore is a diagnosis of exclusion. Although cerebrospinal fluid examination may be normal, an electroencephalogram often shows bilateral temporal slowing. Histopathology demonstrates inflammatory infiltrates of the hippocampus and medial temporal lobes.

Bulbar and brain stem encephalitis can also present with cognitive and memory deficits that are accompanied by vertigo, nystagmus, ataxia, dysphagia, ophthalmoplegia, and extensor plantar reflexes. Subacute cerebellar degeneration often presents with symmetrical ataxia of the arms and legs, dysarthria, diploplia, vertigo, and occasionally nystagmus. Dementia, similar to subcortical dementia, is often an associated finding. Cerebellar degeneration occurs most commonly in patients with ovarian or lung cancer. The syndrome is unfortunately progressive and relenting. Cerebrospinal fluid examination is characterized by increased protein and lymphocytes. Some laboratories have the capacity to detect antineuronal antibodies in the serum of patients with these paraneoplastic neurological syndromes (Anderson et al. 1987).

Table 2–5.   Paraneoplastic syndromes

Brain and cranial nerves
  Limbic encephalitis
  Subacute cerebellar degeneration
  Opsoclonus-myoclonus
  Brain stem encephalitis
  Optic neuritis
  Retinal degeneration
Spinal cord
  Necrotizing myelopathy
Dorsal root ganglia
Peripheral nerve
  Sensorimotor neuropathies
  Guillain-Barré polyradiculoneuropathy
Neuromuscular junction and muscle
  Eaton-Lambert syndrome
  Myasthenic syndrome myopathies
  Cachexia
  Carcinoid myotonias

Medications. Tricyclic antidepressants (e.g., amitriptyline and imipramine), neuroleptic and antiemetic drugs (e.g., chlorpromazine and prochlorperazine), and antihistamines (e.g., diphenhydramine and hydroxyzine) have potent anticholinergic side effects. An "atropine psychosis" or delirium characterized by restlessness, agitation, tachycardia, tachypnea, and hallucinations can occur in patients who are on multiple anticholinergic drugs or who may be vulnerable due to metabolic compromise or advanced age. Narcotic analgesics can also precipitate neuropsychiatric symptoms ranging from oversedation and disinhibition to agitation and delirium. Prominent among the psychiatric symptoms patients experience with narcotic analgesics are illusions or visual hallucinations.

Acyclovir (an antiviral medication used in herpetic infections), when given intravenously, can cause a severe, often treatment-resistant delirium that can be accompanied by tingling of the extremities and tinnitus (Wade and Meyers 1990). The methyl ester form of amphotericin, a powerful antifungal agent, can cause dementia-like symptoms when the accumulated dose reaches more than 9.8 grams (Ellis et al. 1982). Several other antibiotics commonly used in cancer settings have neuropsychiatric side effects. Metronidazole (Flagyl), widely used intravenously in the treatment of infection in patients with cancer or acquired immunodeficiency syndrome (AIDS), can cause encephalopathy, seizures, and cerebellar ataxia when given in high doses (Bailes et al. 1983). Ciprofloxacin (Cipro), a commonly prescribed fluoroquinolone, can cause delirium as well as seizures (Slavich et al. 1989). Cimetidine, a commonly used histamine, subtype 2 (H_2), blocker that inhibits gastric secretions, can produce a florid delirium. Severely medically ill cancer patients, elderly patients who may be physically compromised, and patients on multiple medications with CNS side effects are particularly vulnerable.

Management of Organic Mental Disorders in Cancer Patients

Initially the psychiatric consultant must assess the type and degree of behavioral symptomatology present in the cancer patient with an organic mental disorder such as delirium (Table 2–6). If the change is insidious or mild, there is often more opportunity to gather history and elucidate etiologic factors. If the patient is agitated to the point where his or her own safety or the safety of visitors or staff is threatened, rapid intervention is necessary. Prompt recognition of a mild delirious state can help avoid later emergent situations. Tables 2–7 and 2–8 summarize different schema for the treatment of organic mental disorders in cancer patients. An important second step in the treatment of delirious patients is staff education in the early recognition and management of organic mental disorders.

Management of Mild Organic Mental Disorders

Management of organic mental disorders in cancer patients begins with determination of the underlying etiology. Physical signs and symptoms noted in the chart and by staff often suggest the diagnosis and possible causes. Laboratory data can confirm physical findings or reveal new information. If CNS infection or hemorrhage is suspected, a lumbar puncture (with fluid sent for immediate cell count, glucose, and protein) can be diagnostic. An electroencephalogram may show a pattern of generalized slowing, but does not usually help determine the etiology of confusional states. CT scans of the head with contrast medium can help disclose structural abnormalities or hemorrhage. Magnetic resonance imaging (MRI) scans are more likely to detect more subtle

Table 2–6.   Behavioral symptomatology of delirium in cancer patients

Early symptoms

    Change in sleep patterns; restlessness and transient periods of disorientation

    Increased irritability; anger

    Withdrawal; refusal to talk to staff or relatives

    Forgetfulness that was not previously present

Late symptoms

    Refusal to cooperate with reasonable requests

    Anger, swearing, shouting, and abusive or physical outbursts

    Demanding to go home; pacing the corridor

    Illusions: misidentifying staff; visual and sensory clues

    Delusions: misinterpreting events, usually paranoid in nature; fears of being harmed or poisoned by chemotherapy

    Hallucinations: visual or auditory

changes such as those caused by carcinomatous meningitis.

Manipulation of the environment, judicious use of neuroleptic medications, and adequate monitoring of the patient's course are essential in the management of mild organic mental disorders. Quiet surroundings, well lit during the day and with a soft night-light help avoid the "sundowning" phenomenon at night. Short frequent contacts with family members and staff who reinforce hospital routines and offer clear explanations help reassure the patient and compensate for forgetfulness. Reminders of location, day, time, and outside events help distract patients from dwelling on their own internal thoughts, hallucinations, or delusions and direct them toward appropriate orientation.

Antipsychotic medications given orally are the preferred medications to use in mild organic mental disorders. Benzodiazepines, sedative-hypnotics, or barbiturates may be effective over the first few hours or days, but they may make organic mental disorders worse as active metabolites can accumulate and worsen the patient's confusion. Antihistamines and anticholinergic drugs can sometimes exacerbate a delirium. A neuroleptic drug such as haloperidol is the drug of choice in treating delirium and other organic mental disorders. Haloperidol's high-potency formula has minimal effect on the autonomic nervous system so it produces less orthostatic hypotension and tachycardia. It is available in tablet, liquid concentrate, or parenteral form and has been safely used intramuscularly and intravenously. Initial doses of 0.5 mg once or twice daily can offer sedation and comfort while the cause(s) of behavioral change are sought. Other dopamine-blocking antipsychotic agents can be used in low doses as well (e.g., thioridazine 10 mg, chlorpromazine 10 mg, trifluoperazine 1 mg, and perphenazine 2 mg). Use of low-dose regimens of neuroleptic minimizes the risk of extrapyramidal reactions, such as dystonia, akathisia, and drug-induced parkinsonism. Intramuscular doses should be avoided in patients who are thrombocytopenic from leukemia or from chemotherapy effects.

Table 2–7. Management of mild organic mental disorders

Prompt recognition and diagnosis
Environmental changes to ensure safety
Pharmacological sedation
Possible one-to-one companion
Adequate monitoring

Once the clinician has initiated treatment, frequent follow-up visits help keep medication use to a minimal but effective dose. Adequate recording of patient response and results of the workup through frequent progress notes (noting time) help alert staff of the patient's course. Explanations to the patient and family by staff and the consultant can alleviate a good deal of distress. The following case example illustrates the evolution over time of organic mental disorders in cancer patients:

Case 3

Ms. E, a 73-year-old white woman with lymphoma but no significant medical or psychiatric history, received as treatment cyclophosphamide, doxorubicin, vincristine, and prednisone. She was in complete remission for 6 months when her family noticed that she "no longer seemed like herself." She had lost about 15 lb over the preceding month because she "didn't care to eat" and had not been sleeping through the night but had begun to take daytime naps. She continued to take her dog for his daily walks, but stopped showing interest in television and the newspaper.

Ms. E's initial physical examination did not show any abnormalities. A complete blood count, electrolytes, thyroid function tests, and CT scan of the head with contrast were of little diagnostic help. On mental status examination she was alert and oriented to person, place, and time. She appeared depressed and showed psychomotor slowing. Her affect was blunted. She showed some cognitive and memory

Table 2–8.   Management of severe organic mental disorders

Prompt recognition and diagnosis

Review of all previous blood work and medications

Immediate examination of blood work: complete blood count, electrolytes, and arterial blood gases

Safe environment

One-to-one nurse or companion

Pharmacological sedation

Physical restraint

Adequate monitoring on *all* shifts

Neurology consultation when necessary

deficits: she could follow simple and complex commands; she knew the president, vice president, city, and mayor; but she showed little interest and could not describe recent current events. Her ability to spell, calculate, and repeat a series of numbers was impaired. However, her family reported that she had not been able to perform these functions the year before. She thought that she "might as well be dead, since this is no way to live" but denied suicidal intent. She was initially prescribed lorazepam 1 mg po every 8 hours while the workup was being completed. Although the lorazepam provided some initial sedation, Ms. E became more agitated and developed visual hallucinations. Benzodiazepines were stopped. A switch to nortriptyline, initially at 50 mg, afforded some relief of symptoms. She was eating more and sleeping better at night.

Within a month, Ms. E developed ptosis of her left eye. The "back discomfort" she had been experiencing since the start of her chemotherapy worsened. She began to mutter to herself and misidentify her family members, and she became progressively weaker and confused. Her serum lactic dehydrogenase (LDH) rose from 118 to 475 units and she developed cervical, axillary, and inguinal lymphadenopathy. Subsequent neurological workup revealed lymphomatous meningitis. The nortriptyline was stopped, and haloperidol was begun at 1 mg bid and raised up to 2 mg tid. Intravenous fluids were given to prevent dehydration and plans for terminal care were made. She was less distressed by day-to-day events, less confused, and reported that she "knew she wouldn't make it."

Management of Severe Organic Mental Disorders

Severe agitation from an organic mental disorder in the oncology treatment setting requires prompt recognition and rapid intervention (Table 2–8). Patients are almost always too physically ill to be transferred to psychiatric units, so safety precautions and pharmacological interventions must be adapted to the oncology unit or medical-surgical ward. Confused or belligerent patients who misinterpret events, hallucinate, or are delusional may refuse care or attempt to suddenly leave the hospital. Containing such patients becomes a collaborative effort of the medical, nursing, and security staffs who can be taught about treatment techniques before the occasion arises when they are needed.

Such patients should be moved to a quiet but visible area on the unit and stay in their rooms, out of reach of potentially dangerous objects. A familiar staff member with whom the patient has demonstrated some trust *before* the current incident is often helpful. Oral liquid concentrate forms of haloperidol, thioridazine, or chlorpromazine should be offered because their absorption is fast. If this is inadvisable (i.e., the patient is to receive nothing by mouth, has an upper gastrointestinal obstruction or malabsorption, or refuses), parenteral medication should be considered, avoiding intramuscular injection because of thrombocytopenia. The minimal effective dose should be used and titrated against sedation and autonomic and extrapyramidal side effects. Haloperidol can be given intravenously, (0.5 mg to 2 mg) at 1 mg per minute and repeated every 30 minutes if the agitation is severe. Other authors (e.g., Adams 1988) have advocated the use of higher doses of haloperidol in combination with lorazepam in acute emergencies. The addition of intravenous lorazepam 0.5–2 mg adds to the sedation produced by haloperidol and may in fact reduce the risk of extrapyramidal side effects. Typically, patients are maintained on a regimen of haloperidol, either orally or intravenously, that is equivalent to one-half or two-thirds of the dose required to calm the patient over the initial 24 hours of treatment. Many clinicians prefer to give this maintenance dose in a twice- or three-times-daily regimen.

If pharmacological sedation is inadequate, physical restraint must be temporarily used to ensure safety and prevent self-harm. The application of physical restraints should be directed by a staff member trained to do so safely. Loosely applied cotton padding and soft gauze can be used, provided the patient does not struggle if thrombocytopenic. Limb restraints can prevent the patient from pulling at urinary or intravenous catheters. A "posey" vest confines the patient to bed, but leaves the arms and hands with complete mobility and will not protect catheters from being dislodged. Commercially made mesh sheets restrict arm movements and allow proper ventilation for a patient who is dehydrated or febrile.

Restraints should be used until adequate sedation is achieved. A one-to-one companion to monitor patient needs and level of sedation can help keep the use of restraints to a minimum. Again, with a severely agitated patient, staff and family education provides extra support during such stressful events and encourages compliance. Treatment of organic mental disorders calls on the resources of the whole health care team to provide an adequate workup, correction of etiologic factors, and comfort care techniques simultaneously. Such a challenge is a vital part of modern cancer treatment.

Summary

In this chapter, we reviewed the definition, characteristics, and prevalence of organic mental disorders commonly seen in cancer. Early symptoms and signs are reviewed, as well as those of severe delirium, accompanied by psychotic behavior endangering self and others. Guidelines for managing the delirious cancer patient are outlined, using pharmacological interventions, and environmental manipulation.

References

Adams F: Neuropsychiatric evaluation and treatment of delirium in cancer patients. Adv Psychosom Med 18:26–36, 1988

Adams F, Quesada JR, Gutterman JU: Neuropsychiatric manifestations of human leukocyte interferon therapy in patients with cancer. JAMA 252:938–941, 1984

American Psychiatric Association: Diagnostic and Statistical Manual of Mental Disorders, 3rd Edition, Revised. Washington, DC, American Psychiatric Association, 1987

Anderson NE, Cunningham JM, Posner JB: Autoimmune pathogenesis of paraneoplastic neurologic syndromes. CRC Critical Reviews in Neurobiology 3:245–299, 1987

Bailes J, Willis J, Priebe C, et al: Encephalopathy with metronidazole in a child. Am J Dis Child 37:290–291, 1983

Boston Collaborative Drug Surveillance Program: Acute adverse reactions to prednisone in relation to dosage. Clin Pharmacol Ther 13:694–698, 1972

Breitbart WB: Endocrine-related psychiatric disorders, in Handbook of Psychooncology: Psychological Care of the Patient With Cancer. Edited by Holland JC, Rowland JH. New York, Oxford University Press, 1989, pp 356–366

Caincross JG: Effects of cancer on the nervous system, in Oncologic Therapeutics 1989/90. Edited by Wittes RE. Philadelphia, PA, JB Lippincott, 1989, pp 610–613

DeAngelis LM, Delattre J, Posner JB: Radiation-induced dementia in patients cured of brain metastases. Neurology 39:789–796, 1989

Denicoff KD, Rubinow DR, Papa MZ, et al: The neuropsychiatric effects of treatment with interleukin-2 and lymphokine-activated killer cells. Ann Intern Med 107:293-300, 1987

Derogatis LR, Morrow GR, Fetting J, et al: The prevalence of psychiatric disorders. JAMA 249:751–757, 1983

Ellis WG, Sobel RA, Nielsen SL: Leukencephalopathy in patients treated with amphotericin B methylester. J Infect Dis 146:125–137, 1982

Feinberg WM, Swenson MR: Cerebrovascular complications of L-asparaginase therapy. Neurology 38:127–133, 1988

Fleishman SB, Lesko LM: Delirium and dementia, in Handbook of Psychooncology: Psychological Care of the Patient With Cancer. Edited by Holland JC, Rowland JH. New York, Oxford University Press, 1989, pp 342–355

Gilbey ED, Rees LH, Bondy PK: Biology and characterization of human tumors, in Advances in Tumor Prevention, Detection and Characterization, Vol 3: Proceedings of the Sixth International Symposium. Edited by Davisco M, Malroni C. New York, Elsevier, 1975, pp 99–106

Hall RCW, Popkin MK, Stickney SK, et al: Presentation of steroid psychoses. J Nerv Ment Dis 167:229–236, 1979

Haskett RF: Diagnostic categorization of psychiatric disturbance in Cushing's syndrome. Am J Psychiatry 142:911–916, 1985

Holland J, Fasaniello S, Ohnuma T: Psychiatric symptoms associated with L-asparaginase administration. J Psychiatr Res 10:105–113, 1974

Kaplan RS, Wiernik PH: Neurotoxicity of antineoplastic drugs. Semin Oncol 9:103–130, 1983

Legha SS: Vincristine neurotoxicity. Medical Toxicology 1:421-427, 1986

Levine PM, Silverfarb PM, Lipowski ZJ: Mental disorders in cancer patients: a study of 100 psychiatric referrals. Cancer 42:1385–1391, 1978

Lipowski ZJ: Delirium (acute confusional states). JAMA 285:1789–1792, 1987

Lipowski ZJ: Organic mental disorders and DSM-IV. Am J Psychiatry 147:947–949, 1990

Liston EH: Diagnosis and management of delirium in the elderly. Psychiatric Annals 14:109–118, 1984

Major LF, Brown GL, Wilson WP: Carcinoid and psychiatric symptoms. Southern Medical Journal 66:787–789, 1973

Massie MJ, Holland JC, Glass E: Delirium in terminally ill cancer patients. Am J Psychiatry 140:1048–1050, 1983

Matzen TA, Martin RL: Magnesium deficiency psychosis induced by cancer chemotherapy. Biol Psychiatry 20:788–791, 1985

Mundy GR, Martin JT: Hypercalcemia of malignancy: pathogenesis and management. Metabolism 31:1247–1277, 1982

Patchell RA, Posner JB: Neurologic complications of carcinoid. Neurology 36:745–749, 1986

Patchell RA, Posner JB: Cancer and the nervous system, in Handbook of Psychooncology: Psychological Care of the Patient With Cancer. Edited by Holland JC, Rowland JH. New York, Oxford University Press, 1989, pp 327–341

Phillips PC, Dhawan V, Strother SC, et al: Reduced cerebral glucose metabolism and increased brain capillary permeability following high-dose methotrexate chemotherapy: a positron emission tomographic study. Ann Neurol

21:59–63, 1987

Posner JB: Neurologic complications of systemic cancer. Dis Mon 25:1–60, 1978

Posner JB: Delirium and exogenous metabolic brain disease, in Cecil Textbook of Medicine, 15th Edition. Edited by Beeson PB, McDermolt W, Wyngaarden JB. Philadelphia, PA, WB Saunders, 1979, pp 644–651

Posner JB: Nonmetastatic effects of cancer on the nervous system, in Cecil Textbook of Medicine, 18th Edition. Edited by Wyngaarden JB, Smith LH. Philadelphia, PA, WB Saunders, 1988, pp 1104–1107

Quesada JR, Talpaz M, Rios A, et al: Clinical toxicity of interferons in cancer patients: a review. J Clin Oncol 4:234–243, 1986

Sachs W: Disorders of glucose metabolism in brain dysfunction, in Biology of Brain Dysfunction. Edited by Guall GE. New York, Plenum, 1973, p 143–153

Sandifer MG: Hyponatremia due to psychotropic drugs. J Clin Psychiatry 44:301–303, 1983

Schilsky RL, Anderson T: Hypomagesemia and renal magesium wasting in patients receiving cisplatin. Ann Intern Med 90:929–939, 1979

Seymour DJ, Henschke RD, Cape RD, et al: Acute confusional states and dementia in the elderly: the role of dehydration/volume depletion, physical illness and age. Age Ageing 9:137–146, 1980

Sheline GE: Irradiation injury of the human brain: a review of clinical experience, in Radiation Damage to the Nervous System. Edited by Gilbert J, Kagan AR. New York, Raven, 1980, pp 39–58

Silberfarb PM, Oxman TE: The effect of cancer therapies on the central nervous system. Adv Psychosom Med 18:13–25, 1988

Slavich EL, Gleffe RF, Haas EJ: Grandmal epileptic seizures during ciprofloxacin therapy. JAMA 261:558–559, 1989

Smith KC, Barigh J, Corren J, et al: Psychiatric disturbance in endocrinologic disease. Psychosom Med 34:69–86, 1972

Stiefel FC, Breitbart WS, Holland JC: Corticosteroids in cancer: neuropsychiatric complications. Cancer Invest 7:479–491, 1989

Taylor JW: Depression in thyrotoxicosis. Am J Psychiatry 132:552–553, 1973

Touks CM: Mental illness in hypothyroid patients. Br J Psychiatry 110:706–710, 1974

Tucker G, Popkin M, Caine E, et al: Reorganizing the "organic" disorders. Hosp Community Psychiatry 41:722–724, 1990

Wade JC, Meyers JD: Neurologic symptoms associated with parenteral acyclovir treatment after marrow transplantation. Ann Intern Med 98:921–925, 1990

Young DF, Posner JB: Nervous system toxicity of the chemotherapeutic agents, in Handbook of Clinical Neurology, Vol 39: Neurologic Manifestations of Systemic Diseases, Part II. Edited by Viken PJ, Bruyn GW. New York, Elsevier Biomedical Press, 1980, pp 92–129

Chapter 3

Psychiatric Approaches to Cancer Pain Management

William Breitbart, M.D.
Steven D. Passik, Ph.D.

*C*ancer pain management requires a multidisciplinary approach, enlisting expertise from a wide variety of clinical specialties including neurology, neurosurgery, anesthesiology, and rehabilitation medicine (Foley 1975, 1985). Psychiatric involvement in the treatment of cancer patients with pain has now also become an integral part of such a comprehensive approach (Breitbart 1989; Massie and Holland 1987). Psychological variables such as the meaning of pain, perceptions of control, fear of death, depressed mood, and hopelessness are recognized as contributing to the cancer pain experience (Ahles et al. 1983; Bond 1979; Spiegel and Bloom 1983a). When the International Association for the Study of Pain (Merskey 1986) defined pain as "an unpleasant sensory and emotional experience," it recognized that pain is not simply a somatic nociceptive event, but rather a complex psychological one involving nociception, pain perception, and pain expression (Lindblom et al. 1986; Melzack and Wall 1983).

Multidimensional Concept of Cancer Pain

The interaction of cognitive, emotional, socioenvironmental, and nociceptive aspects of cancer pain shown in Figure 3–1 illustrates the multidimensional nature of cancer pain and suggests a model for multimodal intervention (Breitbart and Holland 1990). The challenge of untangling and addressing both the physical and the psychological issues involved in cancer pain is essential to developing rational and effective management strategies. Psychosocial therapies directed primarily at psychological variables have profound impact on nociception, whereas somatic therapies directed at nociception have beneficial effects on the psychological aspects of cancer pain. Ideally such somatic and psychosocial therapies are used simultaneously in the multidisciplinary approach to cancer pain management (Breitbart 1989).

Psychological Variables and Cancer Pain

The magnitude of the problem is significant, with about 15% of patients with localized disease and between 60% and 90% of those with advanced cancer reporting debilitating pain (Cleeland 1984; Daut and Cleeland 1982; Foley 1975; Kanner and Foley 1981; Twycross and Lack 1983). Pain has profound effects on psychological distress in cancer patients, and psychological factors such as anxiety, depression,

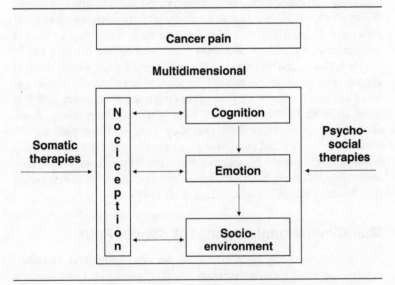

Figure 3–1.   Multidimensional nature of cancer pain. (Reprinted with permission from Breitbart W, Holland J: "Psychiatric Aspects of Cancer Pain," in *Advances in Pain Research and Therapy,* Vol 16. Edited by Foley KM, Bonica JJ, Ventafridda V. New York, Raven, 1990, pp. 73–87.)

and the meaning of pain can intensify cancer pain experience. Daut and Cleeland (1982) showed that cancer patients who attribute a new pain to an unrelated benign cause report less interference with their activity and pleasure than do cancer patients who believe that their pain represents progression of disease. Spiegel and Bloom (1983a) found that women with metastatic breast cancer experienced more intense pain if they believed their pain represented spread of their cancer and if they were depressed. Beliefs about the meaning of pain and the presence of a mood disturbance are better predictors of level of pain than is the site of metastasis. Measures of emotional disturbance have been reported to be predictors of pain in late stages of cancer, and cancer patients with less anxiety and depression were less likely to report pain (Bond 1973; Bond and Pearson 1969; McKegney et al. 1981).

All too frequently, however, psychological variables are proposed to explain continued pain or lack of response to therapy when in fact medical factors have not been adequately appreciated. Often, the psychiatrist is the last physician to consult on a cancer patient with pain and in that role must be vigilant that an accurate pain diagnosis is made and be able to assess the adequacy of the medical analgesic management provided. Psychological distress in patients with pain from cancer must initially be assumed to be the consequence of uncontrolled pain. Personality factors may be quite distorted by the presence of pain, and relief of pain often results in the disappearance of a perceived psychiatric disorder (Cleeland 1984; Marks and Sachar 1973).

Psychiatric Disorders and Cancer Pain

There is an increased frequency of psychiatric disorders found among cancer patients with pain. In the Psychosocial Collaborative Oncology Group Study (Derogatis et al. 1983) on the prevalence of psychiatric disorders in cancer patients, of the 101 patients who received a psychiatric diagnosis, 39% reported significant pain, whereas only 19% of the 114 patients without a psychiatric diagnosis had significant pain (Table 3–1). The psychiatric disorders seen among cancer patients with pain primarily included adjustment disorder with depressed or anxious mood, and major depression. This finding of increased frequency of psychiatric disturbance in cancer pain patients has been reported by others including Ahles et al. (1983) and Woodforde and Fielding (1970).

Epidural spinal cord compression (ESCC) is a common neurological complication of systemic cancer that occurs in 5%–10% of patients with cancer and can often present with severe pain. These patients are routinely treated with a combination of high-dose dexamethasone and radiotherapy. Patients who receive this high-dose regimen are exposed to as much as 96 mg per day of dexamethasone for up to 1 week and continue on a tapering course for up to 3 or 4 weeks. Stiefel et al. (1989) recently described the psychiatric complications seen among cancer patients undergoing such treatment for ESCC: 22% of 50 patients with ESCC were diagnosed as having a major depressive syndrome compared to 4% in the comparison group (*n* = 50). Also, delirium was much more common in the dexamethasone-treated patients with ESCC, with

Table 3–1.   Rates of DSM-III psychiatric disorders and prevalence of pain observed in 215 cancer patients from three cancer centers

Diagnostic category	Diagnostic class		Percentage of psychiatric diagnoses	Number with significant pain[a]	
	n	%		*n*	%
Adjustment disorders	69	32	68		
Major affective disorders	13	6	13		
Organic mental disorders	8	4	8		
Personality disorders	7	3	7		
Anxiety disorders	4	2	4		
Total with psychiatric diagnosis	101	47		39	39
Total with no psychiatric diagnosis	114	53		21	19
Total patient population	215	100		60	28

[a]Score greater than 50 millimeters on a 100-millimeter visual analogue scale for pain severity.
Source.   Reprinted with from Breitbart W, Holland J: "Psychiatric Aspects of Cancer Pain," in *Advances in Pain Research and Therapy,* Vol. 16. Edited by Foley KM, Bonica JJ, Ventrafridda V. New York, Raven, 1990, p. 76. (Data adapted from Deragotis LR, Morrow GR, Getting J, et al: "The Prevalence of Psychiatric Disorders Among Cancer Patients." *JAMA* 249:751–757, 1983.) Used with permission.

24% diagnosed as having delirium during the course of treatment versus only 10% in the comparison group.

Cancer patients with advanced disease are a particularly vulnerable group. The incidence of pain, depression, and delirium increases with greater debilitation and advanced stages of illness (Bukberg et al. 1984). Approximately 25% of all cancer patients experience severe depressive symptoms, with the prevalence increasing to 77% among those with advanced illness. The prevalence of organic mental disorders (delirium) among cancer patients requiring psychiatric consultation has been found to range from 25% to 40% and to be as high as 85% during the terminal stages of illness (Massie et al. 1983). Narcotic analgesics, such as meperidine, levorphanol, and morphine sulfate, can cause confusional states particularly in elderly and terminally ill patients (Bruera et al. 1989b). The following case example illustrates how depression can complicate cancer pain management:

Case 1

Ms. F, a 68-year-old woman with breast cancer widely metastatic to bone, was admitted to the hospital for pain control. On admission, she was screaming in pain and repeatedly demanded, "Kill me, kill me, put me out of my misery." Her repeated requests for euthanasia, despite attempts to control pain with opioid analgesics, prompted a psychiatric consultation. She was put on a regimen of high-dose morphine and nonsteroidal anti-inflammatory drugs, but she continued to report pain intensity of 8 on a visual analogue scale (VAS) of 0 to 10.

On interviewing Ms. F, the consultant learned that she had a history of recurrent major depressions that had responded to tricyclic antidepressants (TCAs) in the past. She presently exhibited many of the signs and symptoms of major depression including hopelessness, helplessness, worthlessness, guilt, and suicidal ideation. She also had numerous neurovegetative signs such as insomnia, listlessness, and fatigue, but it was unclear whether these were depressive indicators or the result of pain and advanced cancer. Her family indicated that she appeared the way she had when depressed in the past, except for the presence of the severe pain. Ms. F was placed under one-to-one observation. The consultant recommended nortriptyline starting at 25 mg and rapidly increasing the dose to 100 mg at bedtime. A serum level of 120 ng/dl was achieved. Within several days, her mood improved, as did her sleep. Gradually her suicidal preoccupations and requests for euthanasia remitted. Ms. F's report of pain intensity was markedly decreased with no change in opioid dosage. Several days later, just before discharge, she was questioned about her earlier requests for euthanasia and her suicidal thoughts. She replied, "You should have realized I was severely depressed."

Cancer Pain and Suicide

Uncontrolled pain is a major factor in cancer suicide (Breitbart 1987, 1990). Cancer is perceived by the public as an extremely painful disease compared with other medical conditions; a study (Levin et al. 1985) in Wisconsin revealed that 69% of the public agreed that cancer pain could cause a person to consider suicide. The majority of suicides observed among cancer patients were among those who had severe pain, which was often inadequately controlled or poorly tolerated (Bolund 1985). Although relatively few cancer patients commit suicide, they are at increased risk (Breitbart 1987; Farberow et al. 1963). Patients with advanced illness are at highest risk and are the most likely to have the complications of pain, depression, delirium, and deficit symptoms. Psychiatric disorders are frequently present in hospitalized cancer patients who attempt suicide. A review of the psychiatric consultation data at Memorial Sloan-Kettering Cancer Center showed that one-third of cancer patients who were seen for evaluation of suicide risk received a diagnosis of major depression, approximately one-fifth met criteria for delirium, and more than half were diagnosed as having an adjustment disorder (Breitbart 1987).

Thoughts of suicide probably occur quite frequently, particularly in the setting of advanced cancer, and seem to act as a steam valve for feelings often expressed by patients, such as "If it gets too bad, I always have a way out." It has been our experience working with cancer pain patients that once a trusting and safe relationship develops, patients almost universally reveal that they have had occasionally persistent thoughts of suicide as a means of escaping the threat of being overwhelmed by pain. Recent reports, however, have suggested that suicidal ideation is relatively infrequent in cancer and is limited to those who are significantly depressed. For example, Silberfarb et al. (1980) found that only 3 of 146 breast cancer patients had suicidal thoughts, and none of the 100 cancer patients interviewed in a Finnish study (Achte and Vanhkonen 1971) expressed suicidal thoughts. A study (Brown et al. 1986) conducted at St. Boniface Hospice in Winnipeg,

Canada, demonstrated that only 10 of 44 terminally ill cancer patients were suicidal or desired an early death and all 10 were suffering from clinical depression. At Memorial Sloan-Kettering Cancer Center, suicide risk evaluation accounted for 8.6% of psychiatric consultations, usually requested by staff in response to patients verbalizing suicidal wishes (Breitbart 1987). Among the 71 cancer patients who had suicidal ideation with serious intent, significant pain was a factor for only 30% of them. In striking contrast, virtually all 71 suicidal cancer patients had a psychiatric disorder (mood disturbance or organic mental disorder) at the time of evaluation (Breitbart 1987).

We recently examined the role of cancer pain in suicidal ideation by assessing 185 cancer pain patients involved in ongoing research protocols of the Memorial Sloan-Kettering Cancer Center Pain and Psychiatry Services (Saltzburg et al. 1989). Suicidal ideation occurred in 17% of the study population with the majority reporting suicidal ideation without intent to act. Interestingly, in this population of cancer patients who all had significant pain, suicidal ideation was not directly related to pain intensity but was strongly related to degree of depression and mood disturbance. Pain was related to suicidal ideation indirectly in that patients' perception of poor pain relief was associated with suicidal ideation. Perceptions of pain relief may have more to do with aspects of hopelessness than with pain itself. Pain plays an important role in vulnerability to suicide; however, associated psychological distress and mood disturbance seem to be essential cofactors in raising the risk of suicide in cancer patients. Pain has adverse effects on patients' quality of life and sense of control and impairs the family's ability to provide support. Factors other than pain, such as mood disturbance, delirium, loss of control, and hopelessness, contribute to cancer suicide risk (Breitbart 1990). The following case example illustrates how suicidal ideation, cancer pain, and cognitive status interact:

Case 2

Ms. G, a 43-year-old married woman with advanced ovarian cancer and severe pelvic and abdominal pain, had multiple admissions for intermittent bowel obstructions and pain control. Each admission was precipitated by increasing pain, emotional distress, and threats of suicide. She generally refused psychiatric intervention to evaluate her suicidality. Typically, she would quickly respond to pain control measures and the extra attention and care she received in the hospital. Finally, she agreed to psychiatric consultation during her most recent hospitalization, while still distressed and suicidal. She complained that she "would rather die" than have her activities curtailed by the side effects of her pain medicines. She indicated that, although her pain control was adequate, "spaciness" and sedation isolated her from her family and friends and made her contemplate suicide. She was receiving hydromorphone 4 mg po every 3–4 hours around the clock. On mental status examination, she appeared sedated with slightly slurred speech. Her concentration and attention were poor, as was her short-term memory. The remainder of her mental status examination results were normal. Her psychiatric history was noteworthy for chronic depressed affect, feelings of emptiness, chronic suicidality with several prior suicide attempts, and a chaotic interpersonal life. Her family psychiatric history included a long line of completed suicides in mother, maternal great aunt, grandmother, and sister.

In terms of her current suicidal preoccupations, Ms. G explained that when she was not sedated or cognitively impaired by pain medicines she was able to participate in activities that allowed her to deny the terminal and serious nature of her illness. Side effects that interrupted this means of coping resulted in despair. To escape this intolerable state her thoughts quickly turned to suicide. She had been hoarding pills and intended to overdose. She continued to feel suicidal in the hospital and could not assure the consultant that she could control her self-destructive impulses. She was considered to be at increased risk of suicide and was placed on one-to-one observation.

The consultant recognized the connections between sedation, impaired coping, and suicidality and suggested the use of a psychostimulant to decrease sedation and improve mood. Ms. G was started on methylphenidate 2.5 mg at 8 A.M. and 2.5 mg at noon, which was titrated up to a dose of 10 mg at 8 A.M. and 10 mg at noon. After 4 days on this regimen, Ms. G's mental state improved dramatically. She denied suicidal ideation, felt her mood to be improved, was more hopeful about the future, and was more alert and able to interact with her husband. During this period her pain regimen was unchanged. After discharge, she continued to function well with good pain control, but she developed insomnia. The consultant added trazodone 150 mg at bedtime, which improved her sleep and did not cause daytime sedation. She continued to do well and went on to seek alternative cancer therapies in Mexico.

Assessment Issues in the Treatment of Cancer Pain: Obstacles to Adequate Pain Control

Inadequate management of cancer pain is often due to a lack of ability to properly assess pain in all its dimensions (Breitbart 1989; Foley 1985; Marks and Sachar 1973). All too frequently, psychological variables are proposed to explain continued pain or lack of response to therapy, when in fact medical factors have not been adequately appreciated. (For a review of cancer pain assessment and medical management, see Chapter 8.) Other causes of inadequate cancer pain management include 1) lack of knowledge of current therapeutic approaches, 2) focus on prolonging life and cure versus alleviating suffering, 3) inadequate physician-patient relationship, 4) limited expectations of patients, 5) unavailability of narcotics, 6) fear of respiratory depression, and 7) (most important) fear of addiction.

Fear of addiction affects both patient compliance and physician management of narcotic analgesics leading to undermedication of cancer pain (Charap 1978; Macaluso et al. 1988; Marks and Sachar 1973). Studies (e.g., Kanner and Foley 1981) of the patterns of chronic narcotic analgesic use in patients with cancer have demonstrated that, although tolerance and physical dependence commonly occur, addiction (psychological dependence) is rare and almost never occurs in individuals without a history of drug abuse before cancer illness. Escalation of narcotic analgesic use by cancer patients is usually due to progression of cancer or the development of tolerance. Tolerance means that a larger dose of narcotic analgesic is required to maintain an original analgesic effect. Physical dependence is characterized by the onset of signs and symptoms of withdrawal if the narcotic is suddenly stopped or a narcotic antagonist is administered. Tolerance usually occurs in association with physical dependence but does not imply psychological dependence or addiction. Addiction is not equivalent to physical dependence or tolerance; it is a behavioral pattern of compulsive drug abuse characterized by a craving for the drug and overwhelming involvement in obtaining and using it for effects other than pain relief.

The cancer pain patient with a history of intravenous opioid abuse presents an often unnecessarily difficult management problem. Macaluso et al. (1988) reported on their experience in managing cancer pain in such a population. Of 468 cancer pain inpatients, only 8 (1.7%)

had a history of intravenous drug abuse, but none had been actively abusing drugs in the previous year. All 8 of these patients had inadequate pain control and were intentionally undermedicated because of concern by staff that drug abuse was active or would recur. Adequate pain control was ultimately achieved in these patients by using appropriate analgesic dosages and intense staff education.

The risk of inducing respiratory depression is too often overestimated and can limit appropriate use of narcotic analgesics for pain and symptom control. Bruera et al. (1990) demonstrated that, in a population of terminally ill cancer patients with respiratory failure and dyspnea, administration of subcutaneous morphine actually improved dyspnea without causing a significant deterioration in respiratory function.

The adequacy of cancer pain management can be influenced by the lack of concordance between patient ratings or complaints of their pain and those made by caregivers. Persistent cancer pain is often ascribed to a psychological cause when it does not respond to treatment attempts. In our clinical experience, we have noted that patients who report their pain as "severe" are quite likely to be viewed as having a psychological contribution to their complaints. Staff members' ability to empathize with a patient's pain complaint may be limited by the intensity of the pain complaint. Grossman et al. (1991) found that, although there is a high degree of concordance between patient and caregiver ratings of patient pain intensity at the low and moderate levels, this concordance breaks down at high levels. Thus a clinician's ability to assess a patient's level of pain becomes unreliable once a patient's report of pain intensity rises above 7 on a visual analogue scale of 0 to 10. Physicians must be educated as to the limitations of their ability to objectively assess the severity of a subjective pain experience. Additionally, patient education is often a useful intervention in such cases. Patients are more likely to be believed and adequately treated if they are taught to request pain relief in a nonhysterical, business-like fashion. The following case example illustrates common assessment barriers to adequate cancer pain management:

Case 3

Ms. H, a 70-year-old recently widowed woman, had urethral cancer metastatic to bladder. She was admitted to the urology service for control of intractable pelvic pain. She had recently undergone resection of tumor and removal of her urinary bladder and developed a rectovaginal fistula postoperatively. Surgery to repair the fistula had been performed in the weeks before her readmission for pain control. Biopsies taken during that procedure were negative. She had a magnetic resonance imaging (MRI) scan and a computed tomography (CT) scan of the pelvis in the month before her admission; neither revealed any residual tumor.

Ms. H had severe incident pain deep in her vagina whenever she would turn in bed, sit up, or stand. Rather than risk exacerbating her pain, she resisted staff attempts to mobilize her. She was treated with high doses of opioid analgesics that were ineffective in controlling the episodic pain. In fact, she would be somnolent on these doses of opioid drugs but still would complain of pain on movement. The lack of response to pain control interventions began to frustrate both her and the staff. Ms. H became depressed, tearful, and hopeless. She began to express grief over the death of her husband who she had nursed through a long debilitating illness.

The staff began to view Ms. H as willfully thwarting their attempts to mobilize and discharge her. They viewed her as disease free and cured. They saw her complaints of pain as an expression of grief and her fear of returning to her now empty home. Psychiatric consultation was requested after she reported decreased pain with the administration of a placebo (normal saline injection). The consultant took note of several depressive symptoms in her presentation and agreed with staff that she was suffering with a complicated bereavement.

To alleviate Ms. H's fatigue, sedation, and depressed mood, the consultant recommended a psychostimulant and started supportive psychotherapy to facilitate the grieving process. Pemoline 37.5 mg po bid was started and titrated up to 75 mg bid. The consultant educated staff members as to the lack of diagnostic significance in her response to placebo. Attempts were made to modify analgesic interventions so that they would be most effective for incident pain. Ms. H was switched from a regimen of high-dose oral opioid analgesics around the clock, to a patient-controlled subcutaneous infusion of morphine. Her mood improved and she was eager to leave the hospital but her pain was so intense that it precluded efforts at mobilization. A long period ensued in which the consultant, not entirely convinced that psychological factors alone explained the pain behavior, repeatedly attempted to persuade staff to restudy her pelvic region for recurrent disease. Finally, to everyone's surprise, a plain X ray of the pelvis revealed lytic lesions in the pelvic bone. Ms. H underwent radiation therapy to the region that resulted in diminished pain that could now be well controlled with opioids and nonsteroidal anti-inflammatory drugs. She went on to be discharged.

Psychiatric Management of Cancer Pain

Optimal treatment of cancer pain is multimodal and includes pharmacological, psychotherapeutic, cognitive-behavioral, anesthetic, stimulatory, and rehabilitative approaches. Psychiatric participation in cancer pain management involves the use of psychotherapeutic, cognitive-behavioral, and psychopharmacological interventions.

Psychotherapy and Cancer Pain

The goals of psychotherapy with cancer pain patients are to provide support, knowledge, and skills (Table 3–2). Using short-term supportive psychotherapy based on a crisis intervention model, the therapist provides emotional support, continuity, and information and assists in adaptation to the crisis. The therapist has a role in emphasizing past strengths, supporting previously successful coping strategies, and teaching new coping skills, such as relaxation, cognitive coping, use of analgesics, self-observation, documentation, assertiveness, and com-

Table 3–2.   Psychotherapy and cancer pain

Goals

Support: provide continuity

Knowledge: provide information

Skills: relaxation, cognitive coping, use of analgesics, and communication

Form

Individuals: supportive and/or crisis intervention

Family: patient and family are the unit of concern

Group: share experiences and identify successful coping strategies

Source.   Adapted from Breitbart W, Holland J: "Psychiatric Aspects of Cancer Pain," in *Advances in Pain Research and Therapy,* Vol. 16. Edited by Foley KM, Bonica JJ, Ventafridda V. New York, Raven, 1990, pp. 73–87. Used with permission.

munication skills. Communication skills are of paramount importance for both patient and family, particularly around pain and analgesic issues. The patient and family are the unit of concern and need a more general, long-term, supportive relationship within the health care system, as well as specific psychological approaches dealing with pain that a psychiatrist, psychologist, social worker, or nurse can provide.

Group interventions with individual patients, spouses, couples, and families are a powerful means of sharing experiences and identifying successful coping strategies. Using psychotherapy to diminish symptoms of anxiety and depression, factors that can intensify pain, empirically has beneficial effects on cancer pain experience. Spiegel and Bloom (1983b) demonstrated, in a controlled randomized prospective study, the effect of both supportive group therapy for metastatic breast cancer patients, in general, and the effect of hypnotic pain control exercises, in particular. Their support group focused not on interpersonal processes or self-exploration, but rather on a series of themes related to the practical and existential problems of living with cancer. Patients were divided into two treatment groups and a control group. The treatment patients experienced significantly less pain than did the control patients. Patients in the group that combined a self-hypnosis exercise group showed a slight increase in pain, and patients in the control group showed a large increase in pain.

Although psychotherapy in the cancer pain setting is primarily nonanalytical and focuses on current issues, exploration of reactions to cancer often involve insights into earlier more pervasive life issues. Some patients choose to continue a more exploratory psychotherapy during extended illness-free periods or survivorship. Two new theoretical constructs of interest to psychotherapists working with chronic noncancer pain patients can be helpful in guiding some of the exploratory work that is occasionally appropriate and helpful to cancer pain patients. These constructs, alexithymia and pain as a dissociative symptom (remnant of early-life trauma), have proven to be useful to us in the psychotherapeutic treatment of some of our cancer pain patients. Psychiatric observations of chronic noncancer pain patients may have relevance to a subset of cancer pain patients as the degree of overlap between these two populations has not yet been well studied. For example, Portenoy and Hagen (1990) found in their survey of cancer patients that there was a greater probability of reporting pain due to cancer in patients who had had premorbid noncancer pain.

Alexithymia. The inability to express and articulate emotional experiences—alexithymia—is thought to be a personality trait associated with chronic pain and somatization. Recent research has demonstrated that it is a variable with some utility in the understanding of the cancer pain patient as well. Dalton and Feuerstein (1989), for example, demonstrated that patients who scored high on a measure of alexithymia experienced prolonged and more severe pain than did patients who scored low. The cancer setting is characterized by highly emotionally charged issues revolving around loss, disability, disfigurement, and death (Massie and Holland 1987). Patients are faced with intense emotions that can be threatening or difficult to articulate. Therapists can be quite helpful to alexithymic patients by acknowledging such feelings and allowing for their verbalization. In many instances, the therapist must actually provide the patient with a lexicon for the expression of those feelings (Passik and Wilson 1987). Relatedly, the meaning of pain can determine the amount of pain reported. As Spiegel and Bloom (1983a) described, women with breast cancer who viewed their pain as a signal that their disease had progressed reported more pain than women who ascribed a benign meaning to their pain. Therapists can help to correct misperceptions about pain when appropriate and allow for the open discussion of issues and fears that might prolong or intensify a pain experience.

Pain as a dissociative symptom. As society has become more aware of the staggering prevalence of child abuse, psychiatrists and psychologists have begun to reexamine the role of early-life trauma in the etiology of psychiatric disorders. This increased awareness has led especially to renewed interest in the dissociative disorders and related phenomena (e.g, psychogenic amnesia, fugue, multiple personality disorder, conversion, and posttraumatic stress disorder). Patients with dissociative disorders have a wide variety of transient physical problems such as dysesthesias, anesthesias, and pain (Terr 1991). In the chronic, nonmalignant pain population there has been a recent clinical and empirical acknowledgement of such problems. Patients with chronic pelvic pain and premenstrual syndrome, for example, were found to have an unusually high prevalence of early sexual abuse (Paddison et al. 1990; Walker et al. 1988). The prevalence of such phenomena in the cancer pain population is unknown. However, the cancer setting, with its life-threatening backdrop, toxic and disfiguring treatments, and invasive procedures, can reawaken long dormant traumata in even high-functioning patients with abuse histories. Inquiry into such issues can be essential to the evaluation and treatment of such patients. Not generally a part of a routine psychiatric assessment in the medical setting, the recognition of the need to inquire into these areas requires attentive listening with the "third ear" (Reik 1948). Case 4 illustrates how traumatic events of the past can influence pain complaints:

Case 4

Mr. I, a 30-year-old graduate student with a 10-year history of rhabdomyosarcoma of the abdomen and pelvis, had courageously faced several years of illness that required multiple surgical procedures. So, when he was admitted to the hospital for a second-look laparotomy after a recent course of chemotherapy, his doctors were surprised by his tremendous fear and trepidation and his somewhat hysterical reports of abdominal pain. A preoperative psychiatric consultation was requested. The consultant found him to be highly articulate and intelligent but also highly anxious and labile in his mood. He seemed quite focused on the fact that the doctors were going to "open [him] up" and repeatedly used phrases such as "they're going to see it" and "they're going to look at it" (referring, ostensibly, to his tumor). The initial meeting was largely uneventful, yielding a negative psychiatric history. Mr. I reported that he was having nightmares that he could not remember. A hypnotic was prescribed for sleep.

On returning for the second visit, the consultant found Mr. I generally unchanged. He continued to be emotionally labile, repeatedly used the phrases referred to above, and reported abdominal and pelvic pain. The consultant pointed out to him that he had seemed quite focused on what the doctors were going to see when they looked inside of him and asked what he thought it was that they were going to look at. At this point Mr. I burst into tears. He was inconsolable for several moments, sobbing loudly. He then reported that the previous night he had remembered a traumatic experience from grade school. In that experience, he (a typically shy and withdrawn youngster) had confessed his attraction to a female classmate. In a cruel prank, the young girl arranged to meet the patient in a "private" spot for a rendezvous having arranged for her female classmates to be hiding in that location. The girl seduced him into taking off his pants, only to have all of her classmates come out of hiding. He was humiliated. After an emotional abreaction the patient was calm, and his complaints of pain ceased.

Cognitive-Behavioral Techniques

Cognitive-behavioral techniques useful in cancer pain (Table 3–3) include passive relaxation with mental imagery, cognitive distraction

Table 3–3. Cognitive-behavioral techniques used by cancer pain patients

Psychoeducation
    Preparatory information
    Self-monitoring
Relaxation
    Passive breathing
    Progressive muscle relaxation
Distraction
    Focusing
    Controlled mental imagery
    Cognitive distraction
    Behavioral distraction
Combined techniques (relaxation and distraction)
    Passive-progressive relaxation with mental imagery
    Systematic desensitization
    Meditation
    Hypnosis
    Biofeedback
    Music therapy
Cognitive therapies
    Cognitive distortion
    Cognitive restructuring
Behavioral therapies
    Modeling
    Graded task management
    Contingency management
    Behavioral rehearsal

Source. Adapted from Breitbart W, Holland J: "Psychiatric Aspects of Cancer Pain," in *Advances in Pain Research and Therapy,* Vol. 16. Edited by Foley KM, Bonica JJ, Ventafridda V. New York, Raven, 1990, pp. 73–87. Used with permission.

or focusing, progressive muscle relaxation, biofeedback, hypnosis, and music therapy (Cleeland 1987; Cleeland and Tearnan 1986; Fishman and Loscalzo 1987). Such behavioral interventions are effective in the control of both chronic cancer pain and acute procedure-related pain. The goal of treatment is to guide the patient toward a sense of control over pain. Some techniques are primarily cognitive in nature, focusing on perceptual and thought processes, and others are directed at modifying patterns of behavior that help cancer patients cope with pain (see Chapter 4).

Behavioral techniques include methods of modifying physiological pain reactions, respondent pain behaviors, and operant pain behaviors. The most fundamental technique is self-monitoring. The development of the ability to monitor one's behaviors allows a person to notice dysfunctional reactions and learn to control them. Systematic desensitization is useful in extinguishing anticipatory anxiety that leads to avoidant behaviors and in remobilizing inactive patients. Graded-task assignment is essentially systematic desensitization as it is applied to patients who are encouraged to take small steps gradually so as to perform activities more readily. Contingency management is a method of reinforcing "well" behaviors only, thus modifying dysfunctional operant pain behaviors associated with secondary gain (Cleeland 1987; Loscalzo and Jacobsen 1990).

Primarily cognitive techniques for coping with pain are aimed at increasing relaxation and reducing the intensity and distress that are part of the pain experience. Cognitive modification is an approach derived from cognitive therapy for depression or anxiety and is based on how one interprets events and bodily sensation. It is assumed that patients have dysfunctional automatic thoughts that are consistent with underlying assumptions and beliefs. Identifying dysfunctional automatic thoughts and underlying beliefs can allow for a more rational response, thus allowing for restructuring or modification of thought processes or cognition (Fishman and Loscalzo 1987).

Cancer patients are highly motivated to learn and practice these methods, and other cognitive-behavioral techniques (described below), because they are often effective not only in symptoms control, but in restoring a sense of self-control, personal efficacy, and active participation in their care. It is important to note that these techniques must not be used as a substitute for appropriate analgesic management of cancer pain, but rather as part of a comprehensive multimodal approach. The lack of side effects of these techniques make them attractive in the oncology setting as a supplement to already complicated medication regimens. The successful use of these techniques should never lead to the erroneous conclusion that the pain was of psychogenic origin and as such not "real."

The mechanisms by which these cognitive and behavioral techniques relieve pain are not known; however, they all seem to share the elements of relaxation and distraction. Distraction or redirection of attention helps reduce awareness of pain, and relaxation reduces muscle tension and sympathetic arousal (Cleeland 1987). Most cancer patients with pain are appropriate candidates for useful application of these techniques; the clinician, however, should take into account the intensity of pain and the mental clarity of the patient. Ideal candidates have mild to moderate pain and can expect benefit, whereas patients with severe pain can expect limited benefit from psychological interventions unless somatic therapies can lower the level of pain to some degree. Confusional states interfere dramatically with a patient's ability to focus attention and thus limit the usefulness of these techniques (Loscalzo and Jacobsen 1990).

Relaxation and imagery.   Several techniques are used to achieve a mental and physical state of relaxation. Muscular tension, autonomic arousal, and mental distress exacerbate pain (Cleeland 1987; Loscalzo and Jacobsen 1990). Specifically, such relaxation techniques include 1) passive relaxation, focusing attention on sensations of warmth and decreased tension in various parts of the body; 2) progressive muscle relaxation, involving active tensing and relaxing of muscles; and 3) meditation.

Clinically, relaxation techniques are most helpful in managing pain when combined with some distracting or pleasant imagery. The use of distraction or focusing involves control over the focus of attention. One can employ imaginative inattention by picturing oneself on a beach. Mental distraction can be used and is similar to the practice of counting sheep to aid sleep. Keeping oneself busy is a form of behavioral distraction. Imagery (i.e., using one's imagination while in a relaxed state) can be used to transform pain into a warm or cold sensation. One can also imaginatively transform the context of pain (i.e., imagining oneself in battle on the football field instead of the hospital bed). Disassociated somatization can be employed by some patients whereby they imagine that a painful body part is no longer part of their body (Breitbart 1987; Fishman and Loscalzo 1987; Loscalzo and Jacobsen 1990). It is important to note that every patient finds these techniques acceptable, and the therapist must try out a number of approaches to determine which are consistent with the patient's style.

Hypnosis. Hypnosis is efficacious in the treatment of some cancer pain (Barber and Gitelson 1980; Redd et al. 1983; Spiegel 1985; Spiegel and Bloom 1983b). The hypnotic trance is essentially a state of heightened and focused concentration, and thus it can be used to manipulate the perception of pain. The depth of hypnotizability may determine the effectiveness as well as the strategies used during hypnosis. One-third of cancer patients are not hypnotizable, and it is recommended that other techniques be employed for them. Of the two-thirds of patients who are identified as being less, moderately, and highly hypnotizable, three principles underlie the use of hypnosis in controlling pain (Spiegel 1985): 1) use self-hypnosis; 2) relax, do not fight the pain; and 3) use a mental filter to ease the hurt in pain. Patients who are moderately or highly hypnotizable can often alter sensations in a painful area by changing temperature sensation or experiencing tingling. Patients who are hypnotizable to a lesser degree can still use techniques that distract attention, such as concentrating on a mental image of a pleasant scene.

Biofeedback. Fotopoulos et al. (1979) noted significant pain relief in a group of cancer patients who were taught electromyographic (EMG)- and electroencephalographic (EEG)-biofeedback–assisted relaxation. Only 2 of 17 patients were able to maintain analgesia after the treatment ended. A lack of generalization of effect can be a problem with biofeedback techniques. Although physical condition may make a prolonged training period impossible, especially for terminally ill patients, most cancer patients can often use EMG- and temperature-biofeedback techniques for learning relaxation-assisted pain control (Cleeland 1987).

Music therapy. Munro and Mount (1978) have written extensively on the use of music therapy with cancer patients, documenting clinical examples and suggesting mechanisms of action. Music can often capture the focus of attention like no other stimulus and helps patients distract their perception of pain, while expressing themselves in meaningful ways. The following case example illustrates the use of relaxation and imagery in the control of cancer pain:

Case 5

Ms. J, a 42-year-old woman with breast cancer metastatic to bone and the chest wall, experienced restriction of breathing, severe pain, and anxiety. She was referred to psychiatry for help in managing these problems. She was on a regimen of opioid analgesics and nonsteroidal anti-inflammatory agents that resulted in significant reduction in pain. However, residual pain and anxiety remained as clinically important problems. The consultant learned that she was an intensely independent person who experienced a distressing loss of control with the progression of her illness and its encroachment on her ability to breath comfortably. She had practiced meditation in the past and was interested in using such techniques to help manage her current distress.

Ms. J was first taught a simple progressive muscle relaxation exercise that was later combined with a pleasant, distracting image (sitting on the porch of her country home). Later she was able to incorporate a form of dissociative imagery with which she was able to "leave her body" and be pain free for short periods of time, thus breaking the pain cycle. A particularly creative image that she devised and used to her benefit involved imagining that her chest pain was due to a giant bear trap closing on her torso. She would then imagine herself darting into a telephone booth and emerging as "Superwoman," capable of prying open the trap. The use of such imagery relieved pain and anxiety and allowed her to regain a sense of control over her illness.

Psychotropic Adjuvant Analgesic Drugs

Cancer patients with pain have much to gain from the appropriate and maximal use of psychotropic drugs. Psychotropic drugs, particularly the TCAs, are useful as adjuvant analgesics in the pharmacological management of cancer pain. Psychiatrists are often the most experienced in the clinical use of these drugs and so can play an important role in assisting pain control. Table 3–4 lists the various psychotropic medications with analgesic properties, their routes of administration, and their approximate daily doses. These medications not only effect the concomitant anxiety, depression, insomnia, and delirium that can-

Table 3–4. Psychotropic adjuvant analgesic drugs for cancer pain

Drugs (by class)	Trade name	Approximate daily dosage range (mg)	Route
Tricyclic antidepressant			
Amitriptyline	Elavil	10–150	po, im, pr
Nortriptyline	Pamelor	10–50	po
Imipramine	Tofranil	12.5–150	po, im
Desipramine	Norpramin	12.5–150	po
Clomipramine	Anafranil	10–150	po
Doxepin	Sinequan	12.5–150	po, im
Noncyclic antidepressant			
Trazodone	Desyrel	25–300	po
Fluoxetine	Prozac	20–60	po
Paroxetine		40	po
Monoamine oxidase inhibitor			
Phenelzine	Nardil	45–75	po
Amine precursor			
L-Tryptophan		500–3,000	po
Psychostimulant			
Methylphenidate	Ritalin	2.5–20 bid	po
Dextroamphetamine	Dexedrine	2.5–20 bid	po
Phenothiazine			
Fluphenazine	Prolixin	1–3	po, im
Methotrimeprazine	Levoprome	10–20 q6h	im, iv
Butyrophenone			
Haloperidol	Haldol	1–3	po, im, iv
Pimozide	Orap	2–6 bid	po
Antihistamine			
Hydroxyzine	Vistaril	50 q4–6h	po, im, iv
Benzodiazepine			
Alprazolam	Xanax	0.25–2.0 tid	po
Clonazepam	Klonopin	0.5–4 bid	po

Note. po = per oral; im = intramuscular; pr = parenteral; iv = intravenous; q6h = every 6 hours; q4–6h = every 4 to 6 hours; tid = three times a day; bid = two times a day.

Source. Adapted from Breitbart W, Holland J: "Psychiatric Aspects of Cancer Pain," in *Advances in Pain Research and Therapy,* Vol. 16. Edited by Foley KM, Bonica JJ, Ventafridda V. New York, Raven, 1990, pp. 73–87. Used with permission.

cer patients with pain develop, they also have innate analgesic properties of their own.

Antidepressants. The current literature supports the use of antidepressants as adjuvant analgesic agents in the management of a wide
variety of chronic pain syndromes, including cancer pain (Butler 1986;
France 1987; Getto et al. 1987; Magni et al. 1987; Ventafridda et al.
1987; Walsh 1983, 1990). There is substantial evidence that the TCAs,
in particular, are analgesic and useful in the management of chronic
pain syndromes such as postherpetic neuralgia, diabetic neuropathy,
fibromyalgia, headache, and low-back pain.

Amitriptyline is the TCA most studied (and proven effective as an
analgesic) in a large number of clinical trials, addressing a wide variety
of chronic pains (Max et al. 1987, 1988; Pilowsky et al. 1982; Sharav
et al. 1987; Watson et al. 1982). Other TCAs that have been shown to
have efficacy as analgesics include imipramine (Kvindesal et al. 1984;
Sindrup et al. 1989; Young and Clarke 1985), desipramine (Max et al.
1991), nortriptyline (Gomez-Perez et al. 1985), clomipramine (Langohr et al. 1982; Tiegno et al. 1987), and doxepin (Hameroff et al.
1982). Table 3–5 is a compilation of the studies done, both controlled
and uncontrolled, that demonstrated adjuvant analgesic efficacy of
antidepressants for cancer pain. The antidepressants most commonly
used in clinical studies on the management of cancer pain are amitriptyline, imipramine, clomipramine, trazodone, and doxepin (Magni et
al. 1987; Ventafridda et al. 1987; Walsh 1986).

In a placebo-controlled double-blind study of imipramine in
chronic cancer pain, Walsh (1986) demonstrated that imipramine had
analgesic effects independent of its mood effects and was a potent
coanalgesic when used along with morphine. In general, the TCAs are
used in cancer pain as adjuvant analgesics, potentiating the effects of
opioid analgesics, and are rarely used as the primary analgesic (Botney
and Fields 1983; Ventafridda et al. 1987; Walsh 1986). Ventafridda et
al. (1987) reviewed a multicenter clinical experience with antidepressant agents (trazodone and amitriptyline) in the treatment of chronic
cancer pain that included a deafferentation of neuropathic component.
Almost all of their patients were already receiving weak or strong
opioids and experienced improved pain control. A subsequent randomized double-blind study (Ventafridda et al. 1987) showed both amitriptyline and trazodone to have similar therapeutic analgesic efficacy.

Magni et al. (1987) reviewed the use of antidepressants in Italian cancer centers and found that a wide range of antidepressants were used for various cancer pain syndromes, with amitriptyline being the most commonly prescribed. In nearly all cases, antidepressants were used in association with opioids. Good or fair analgesic results were reported in 51% of patients, and the inclusion of all worthwhile responses (e.g., improved sleep) raised the proportion with benefit to 98%.

Table 3–5. Antidepressants for cancer pain

Study	Drug	Efficacy of pain relief (%)
Gebhardt et al. 1969	Clomipramine	67
Adjan 1970	Clomipramine	90
Bernard and Scheuer 1972	Clomipramine plus neuroleptic	87
Adjan 1970	Imipramine	80
Monkemeier and Steffen 1970	Imipramine	75
Barjou 1971	Imipramine	70–80
Deutschmann 1971	Imipramine	80
Hughes et al. 1963	Imipramine	70
Fiorentino 1969[a]	Imipramine	p
Walsh 1986[a]	Imipramine	p
Ventafridda et al. 1987[a]	Amitriptyline vs. trazodone	p / p
Magni et al. 1987	Amitriptyline / Imipramine / Clomipramine / Trazodone / Doxepin	51–98
Breivik and Rennemo 1982	Amitriptyline	67
Bourhis et al. 1978	Amitriptyline / Trimipramine	None / None
Carton et al. 1976	Amitriptyline	70–80
Fernandez et al. 1987[a]	Alprazolam	75

Note. p = drug more effective than placebo.
[a]Controlled study.

The TCAs are effective as adjuvants in cancer pain through a number of mechanisms (Table 3–6), including 1) antidepressant activity (France 1987), 2) potentiation or enhancement of opioid analgesia (Botney and Fields 1983; Malseed and Goldstein 1979; Ventafridda et al. 1990), and 3) direct analgesic effects (Spiegel et al. 1983). Relief of depression in patients with chronic pain has been demonstrated to result in reported pain relief (Bradley 1963); thus the antidepressant effects of the TCAs probably do make a contribution to the analgesic properties of this class of drugs. The TCAs potentiate the analgesic effects of the opioid drugs through direct action on the central nervous system (Botney and Fields 1983) that is likely serotonergically or cholinergically mediated. In addition, the TCAs potentiate the analgesic effects of opioids through a pharmacokinetic mechanism. Desipramine, for instance, will elevate methadone levels in serum (Liu and Wang 1975).

The TCAs have effects on a number of neurotransmitters and their receptors (Charney et al. 1981; Gram 1983); however, it is believed that their activity as potent serotonergic agents (serotonin reuptake blockers) is what mediates their direct, innate analgesic properties (Fields and Basbaum 1984; Gram 1983). Other possible mechanisms of antidepressant analgesic activity include catecholamine effects, adrenergic

Table 3–6.   Possible mechanisms of antidepressant analgesia

Antidepressant activity
Potentiation of opioid effects
   Serotonin and catecholamine
   Pharmacokinetic
   Anticholinergic
Direct analgesic effects
   Serotonin reuptake blockade
   Norepinephrine reuptake blockade
   Opioid receptor binding
   Desensitization of α_2-, and β-adrenergic receptors
   Potentiation of α_1-adrenergic and serotonin receptor agonists
   Decreasing sensitivity of adrenergic receptors on injured nerve
     sprouts
   Inhibiting paroxysmal neuronal discharges
   Adenosinergic effects
   Antihistamine effects

---

and serotonin receptor effects (Gram 1983), adenosinergic effects (Merskey and Hamilton 1989; Salter and Henry 1987), antihistaminic or anticholinergic effects (Gram 1983), and direct neuronal effects such as inhibition of paroxysmal neuronal discharge and decreasing sensitivity of adrenergic receptors on injured nerve sprouts (Devor 1983; Young and Clarke 1985).

The heterocyclic and noncyclic antidepressant drugs such as trazodone, mianserin, and maprotiline and the newer selective serotonin reuptake inhibitors (SSRIs) fluoxetine and paroxetine may also be useful as adjuvant analgesics for cancer patients with pain; however, clinical trials of their efficacy as analgesics have been equivocal. Trazodone has been found to be analgesic in a cancer pain population (Ventafridda et al. 1987); however, a trial for dysesthetic pain in patients with traumatic myelopathy failed to show efficacy (Davidoff et al. 1987). Mianserin (not presently available in the United States) is a potent serotonin reuptake blocker with few adverse side effects, thus making it an attractive choice as an antidepressant or adjuvant analgesic in cancer pain patients (Costa et al. 1985). Maprotiline, a norepinephrine reuptake blocker, demonstrated moderate analgesic properties against clomipramine in a controlled comparison study (Eberhard et al. 1988).

Although the serotonergic properties of the antidepressants are hypothesized to be the primary mechanism of analgesia, clearly, antidepressants with norepinephrinergic properties are useful as well. The serotonin hypothesis of antidepressant analgesia is further complicated by the fact that clinical analgesic studies involving the SSRIs have been equivocal. Fluoxetine is a potent antidepressant (Feighner 1985) that has been shown to have analgesic properties in experimental animal pain models (Hynes et al. 1985). There are no well-controlled studies of fluoxetine as an analgesic for chronic pain; however, several case reports suggest that fluoxetine may be a useful adjuvant analgesic in the management of headache (Diamond and Frietag 1989), fibrositis (Geller 1989), and diabetic neuropathy (Theesen and Marsh 1989). Zimelidine (an SSRI not available in the United States) has not been demonstrated in clinical trials to be consistently effective as an analgesic (Watson and Evans 1985). Paroxetine, soon to be released in the United States, is the first SSRI shown to be a highly effective analgesic in the treatment of neuropathic pain (Sindrup et al. 1990) and may be a useful addition to our armamentarium of adjuvant analgesics for cancer pain. At this point, it is clear that many antidepressants have analgesic properties. There is no definite indication that any one drug is more effective than the others, although the most experience has been accrued with amitriptyline, which remains the drug of first choice.

What is the appropriate dose of TCA when the drug is used as an analgesic and not as an antidepressant? Some researchers (e.g., Sharav et al. 1987) initially advocated a low-dose regimen (10–30 mg) of amitriptyline as being equally analgesic to a high-dose regimen (75–150 mg) of amitriptyline; however, Zitman et al. (1990) demonstrated only modest analgesic results from low-dose amitriptyline. Watson et al. (1984) felt there was a "therapeutic window" (20–100 mg) for the analgesic effects of amitriptyline. More recently, there has been compelling evidence that the therapeutic analgesic effects of amitriptyline are correlated with serum levels just as the antidepressant effects are, and analgesic treatment failure is due to low serum levels (Max et al. 1987, 1988). A high-dose regimen of up to 150 mg of amitriptyline or higher is suggested (Kvindesal 1984; Watson et al. 1984).

As to the time course of onset of the analgesia with antidepressants, there appears to be a biphasic process that occurs. There are immediate or early analgesic effects that occur within hours or days that are probably mediated by inhibition of synaptic reuptake of catecholamines (Botney and Fields 1983; Spiegel et al. 1983; Tiegno et al. 1987). In addition, there are later, longer analgesic effects that peak over a 4- to 6-week period that are likely due to receptor effects of the TCAs (Max et al. 1987, 1988; Pilowsky et al. 1982).

Treatment should be initiated with a small dose and increased slowly (e.g., amitriptyline 10–25 mg at bedtime increased slowly by 10–25 mg every 2 to 4 days towards 150 mg)—especially in debilitated patients—with frequent assessment of pain and side effects until a beneficial effect is achieved. Maximal effect as an adjuvant analgesic may require continuation of drug for 2–6 weeks. When available, serum levels of the antidepressant may also help ensure that therapeutic levels of the drug are being achieved. Both pain and depression in cancer patients often respond to lower doses (25–100 mg) of antidepressant than are usually required in physically healthy patients (100–300 mg), most likely because of impaired metabolism of these drugs. The choice of drug often depends on the side effect profile, existing medical problems, the nature of depressive symptoms if present, and past response to specific antidepressants. Sedating drugs like amitriptyline are helpful when insomnia complicates the presence of pain and depression in a cancer patient. The anticholinergic properties of some of these drugs should also be kept in mind. Occasionally, in patients who have limited analgesic response to a TCA, potentiation of analgesia can be accomplished with the addition of lithium augmentation (Tyler 1974).

Tryptophan, a serotonin precursor, has been used for chronic pain (King 1980; Seltzer et al. 1983) in doses of 2–4 g; however, nausea is a common side effect with higher doses thus limiting usefulness in debilitated cancer patients. Monoamine oxidase inhibitors (MAOIs) are also less useful in the cancer setting because of dietary restrictions and potentially dangerous interactions between MAOIs and narcotics such as meperidine. Among the MAOI drugs available, phenelzine has been shown to have adjuvant analgesic properties in patients with atypical facial pain and migraine (Anthony and Lance 1969; Lascelles 1966). The following case example illustrates the efficacy of a TCA in the management of chemotherapy-induced neuropathic pain:

Case 6

Ms. K, a 46-year-old woman with non-Hodgkin's lymphoma, was on the verge of prematurely terminating chemotherapy for reasons that were unclear to her oncologist. The psychiatric consultant discovered that her reasons for refusing further treatment centered around distress related to a number of unaddressed physical and psychological symptoms. A painful peripheral neuropathy induced by chemotherapy had not been recognized or treated. This resulted in severe insomnia, increasing depression, and agitation. The consultant prescribed amitriptyline, with an initial bedtime dose of 25 mg po. The sedating properties of amitriptyline quickly resulted in improved sleep. The dose was titrated up to 150 mg po at bedtime. At this dose, Ms. K experienced significant pain relief. Her mood improved several days later. A serum amitriptyline level confirmed that a therapeutic level of drug had been reached. With her distress relieved, the patient went on to complete chemotherapy.

Psychostimulants. The psychostimulants dextroamphetamine and methylphenidate are useful antidepressant agents prescribed selectively for medically ill cancer patients with depression (Fernandez et al. 1987b; Katon and Raskind 1980; Kaufmann et al. 1982). Psychostimulants are also useful in diminishing excessive sedation secondary to narcotic analgesics and are potent adjuvant analgesics.

Bruera et al. (1987, 1989a) demonstrated that a regimen of 10 mg methylphenidate with breakfast and 5 mg with lunch significantly decreased sedation and potentiated the analgesic effect of narcotics in patients with cancer pain. Dextroamphetamine has also been reported to have additive analgesic effects when used with morphine in postoperative pain (Forrest et al. 1977). In relatively low doses, psychostimulants stimulate appetite, promote a sense of well-being, and improve feelings of weakness and fatigue in cancer patients. Treatment with dextroamphetamine or methylphenidate usually begins with a dose of 2.5 mg at 8:00 A.M. and at noon. The dosage is slowly increased over several days until a desired effect is achieved or side effects (e.g., overstimulation, anxiety, insomnia, paranoia, and confusion) intervene. Typically a dose greater than 30 mg per day is not necessary, although occasionally patients require up to 60 mg per day.

Patients usually are maintained on methylphenidate for 1–2 months, and approximately two-thirds will be able to be withdrawn from methylphenidate without a recurrence of depressive symptoms. Those who have a recurrence of symptoms can be maintained on a psychostimulant for up to 1 year without significant abuse problems; although, tolerance will develop and adjustment of the dose may be necessary. A strategy we have found useful in treating cancer pain associated with depression is to start a psychostimulant (e.g., starting dose of 2.5 mg of methylphenidate at 8 A.M. and noon) and then to add a TCA after several days to help prolong and potentiate the short effect of the stimulant.

Pemoline is a unique alternative psychostimulant that is chemically unrelated to amphetamine, but may have similar usefulness as an antidepressant and adjuvant analgesic in cancer patients (Breitbart and Mermelstein, in press). Advantages of pemoline as a psychostimulant in cancer pain patients include the lack of abuse potential, the lack of federal regulation through special triplicate prescriptions, the mild sympathomimetic effects, and the fact that it comes in a chewable tablet form that can be absorbed through the buccal mucosa and thus used by cancer patients who have difficulty swallowing or have intestinal obstruction. In our clinical experience, pemoline is as effective as methylphenidate or dextroamphetamine in the treatment of depressive symptoms and in countering the sedating effects of opioid analgesics. There are no studies of pemoline's capacity to potentiate the analgesic properties of opioids. Pemoline can be started at a dose of 18.75 mg in the morning and at noon, and increased gradually over days. Typically patients require 75 mg per day or less. Pemoline should be used with caution in patients with liver impairment, and liver function tests should be monitored periodically with longer-term treatment (Nehra et al. 1990).

Neuroleptics. Methotrimeprazine is a phenothiazine that is equianalgesic to morphine, has none of the opioid effects on gut motility, and probably produces analgesia through α-adrenergic blockade (Beaver et al. 1966). In patients who are opioid tolerant, methotrimeprazine provides an alternative approach in providing analgesia by a nonopioid mechanism. It is a dopamine blocker and so has antiemetic as well an anxiolytic effects. Methotrimeprazine can produce sedation and hypotension and should be given cautiously by slow intravenous infusion. Other phenothiazines such as chlorpromazine and prochlorperazine (Compazine) are useful as antiemetics in cancer patients, but probably have limited use as analgesics (Houde and Wallenstein 1966). Fluphenazine in combination with TCAs has been shown helpful in neuropathic pains (Gomez-Perez et al. 1985). Haloperidol is the drug of choice in the management of delirium or psychoses in cancer patients and has clinical usefulness as a coanalgesic for cancer pain (Maltbie et al. 1979). Pimozide (Orap), a butyrophenone, has been shown to be effective as an analgesic in the management of trigeminal neuralgia at doses of 4–12 mg per day (Lechin et al. 1989).

Anxiolytics. Hydroxyzine is a mild anxiolytic with sedating and analgesic properties that are useful in the anxious cancer patient with pain (Beaver and Feise 1976). This antihistamine has antiemetic activity as well; 100 mg of parenteral hydroxyzine has analgesic activity approaching 8 mg of morphine, and has additive analgesic effects when combined with morphine. Benzodiazepines have not been felt to have specific analgesic properties, although they are potent anxiolytics and anticonvulsants. Some authors have suggested that their anticonvulsant properties make certain benzodiazepine drugs useful in the management of neuropathic pain. Recently, Fernandez et al. (1987a) showed that alprazolam, a unique benzodiazepine with mild antidepressant properties, was a helpful adjuvant analgesic in cancer patients with phantom limb pain or deafferentation (neuropathic) pain. Clonazepam

(Klonopin) may also be useful in the management of lancinating neuropathic pains in the cancer setting and has been reported to be an
effective analgesic for patients with trigeminal neuralgia, headache,
and posttraumatic neuralgia (Caccia 1975; Swerdlow and Cundill
1981).

Summary

The mainstay of pharmacological interventions for cancer pain continues to be the appropriate use of narcotic analgesics. There is, however,
growing awareness and acceptance of the benefits for cancer pain
patients derived from psychiatric contributions to pain control. Unfortunately, cancer patients with pain are most vulnerable to psychiatric
complications of cancer such as depression, anxiety, and delirium. The
clinician who wants to provide comprehensive management of cancer
pain must be familiar with or have available expertise in psychiatric
assessment and intervention in cancer patients. Knowledge of the indications and usefulness of psychotropic drugs in the cancer pain population will be most rewarding, particularly because these drugs are
useful not only in the treatment of psychiatric complications of cancer,
but also as adjuvant analgesic agents in the management of cancer pain.
Psychotherapy and cognitive-behavioral techniques have also been
shown to decrease psychological distress in cancer pain patients, and
provide useful tools for regaining control and reducing cancer pain.
Psychopharmacological, psychotherapeutic, and cognitive-behavioral
interventions are all powerful psychiatric contributions to a multidisciplinary approach in the management of cancer pain.

References

Achte KA, Vanhkonen ML: Cancer and the psych. Omega 2:46–56, 1971
Adjan M: Uber therapeutischen Beeinflussung des Schmerzsymptoms bei un-
    heilboren Tumorkranken. Therapie der Gergenwart 10:1620–1627, 1970
Ahles TA, Blanchard EB, Ruckdeschel JC: The multidimensional nature of
    cancer related pain. Pain 17:277–288, 1983
Anthony M, Lance JW: MAO inhibition in the treatment of migraine. Arch
    Neurol 21:263–264, 1969
Barber J, Gitelson J: Cancer pain: psychological management using hypnosis.
    CA 3:130–136, 1980

Barjou B: Etude du Tofranil sules douleurs en chirugie. Revue Medecin Tours 6:473–482, 1971

Beaver WT, Wallenstein SL, Houde RW, et al: A comparison of the analgesic effect of methotrimeprazine and morphine in patients with cancer. Clin Pharmacol Ther 7:436–446, 1966

Beaver WT, Feise G: Comparison of the analgesic effects of morphine, hydroxyzine and their combination in patients with post-operative pain, in Advances in Pain Research and Therapy. Edited by Bonica JJ, Albe-Fessard. New York, Raven, 1976, pp 533–557

Bernard A, Scheuer H: Action de la clomipramine (Anafranil) sur la douleur des cancers en pathologie cervico-faciale. Journal Francais d'Otorhino-laryngologie 21:723–728, 1972

Bolund C: Suicide and cancer, II: medical and care factors in suicide by cancer patients in Sweden: 1973–1976. Journal of Psychosocical Oncology 3:17–30, 1985

Bond MR: Personality studies in patients with pain secondary to organic disease. J Psychosomatic Res 17:257–263, 1973

Bond MR: Psychological and emotional aspects of cancer pain, in Advances in Pain Research and Therapy, Vol 2. Edited by Bonica JJ, Ventafridda V. New York, Raven, 1979 pp, 81–88

Bond MR, Pearson IB: Psychological aspects of pain in women with advanced cancer of the cervix. J Psychosom Res 13:13–19, 1969

Botney M, Fields HC: Amitriptyline potentiates morphine analgesia by direct action on the central nervous system. Ann Neurol 13:160–164, 1983

Bourhis A, Boudouresue G, Pellet W, et al: Pain, infirmity and psychotropic drugs in oncology. Pain 5:263–274, 1978

Bradley JJ: Severe localized pain associated with the depressive syndrome. Br J Psychiatry 109:741–745, 1963

Breitbart W: Suicide in cancer patients. Oncology 1:49–53, 1987

Breitbart W: Psychiatric management of cancer pain. Cancer 63:2336–2342, 1989

Breitbart W: Cancer pain and suicide, in Advances in Pain Research and Therapy, Vol 16. Edited by Foley KM, Bonica JJ, Ventafridda V. New York, Raven, 1990, pp 399–412

Breitbart W, Holland J: Psychiatric aspects of cancer pain, in Advances in Pain Research and Therapy, Vol 16. Edited by Foley KM, Bonica JJ, Ventafridda V. New York, Raven, 1990, pp 73–87

Breitbart W, Mermelstein H: Pemoline: an alternative psychostimulant in the management of depressive disorders in cancer patients. Psychosomatics (in press)

Breivik H, Rennemo F: Clinical evaluation of combined treatment with methadone and psychotropic drugs in cancer patients. Acta Anaesthesiol

Scand Suppl 74:135–140, 1982

Brown JH, Henteleff P, Barakat S, et al: Is it normal for terminally ill patients to desire death? Am J Psychiatry 143:208–211, 1986

Bruera E, Chadwick S, Brennels C, et al: Methylphenidate associated with narcotics for the treatment of cancer pain. Cancer Treatment Reports 71:67–70, 1987

Bruera E, Brenneis C, Paterson AH, et al: Use of methylphenidate as an adjuvant to narcotic analgesics in patients with advanced cancer. Journal of Pain Symptom Management 4:3–6, 1989a

Bruera E, MacMillan K, Kachin N, et al: The cognitive effects of the administration of narcotics. Pain 39:13–16, 1989b

Bruera E, MacMillan K, Pither J, et al: Effects of morphine on the dyspnea of terminal cancer patients. Journal of Pain Symptom Management 5:341–344, 1990

Bukberg J, Penman D, Holland J: Depression in hospitalized cancer patients. Psychosom Med 43:199–222, 1984

Butler S: Present status of tricyclic antidepressants in chronic pain therapy, in Advances in Pain Research and Therapy, Vol 7. Edited by Benedetti C, Chapman RC, Moricca G. New York, Raven, 1984, pp 173–196

Caccia MR: Clonazepam in facial neuralgia and cluster headache: clinical and electrophysiological study. Eur Neurol 13:560–563, 1975

Carton M, Cabarrot E, Lafforque C: Interest de l'amitriptyline utilisee commee antalgique en cancerologie. Gazette Medecin Francais 83:2375–2378, 1976

Charap AD: The knowledge, attitudes, and experience of medical personnel treating pain in the terminally ill. Mt Sinai J Med 45:561–580, 1978

Charney DS, Meukes DB, Heniuger PR: Receptor sensitivity and the mechanism of action of antidepressant treatment. Arch Gen Psychiatry 38:1160–1180, 1981

Cleeland CS: The impact of pain on the patient with cancer. Cancer 54:2635–2641, 1984

Cleeland CS: Nonpharmacologic management of cancer pain. Journal of Pain and Symptom Control 2:523–528, 1987

Cleeland CS, Tearnan BH: Behavioral control of cancer pain, in Pain Management. Edited by Holzman D, Turk DC. New York, Pergamon, 1986, pp 193–212

Costa D, Mogos I, Toma T: Efficacy and safety of mianserin in the treatment of depression of woman with cancer. Acta Psychiatr Scand 72:85–92, 1985

Dalton JA, Feuerstein M: Fear, alexithymia and cancer pain. Pain 38:159–170, 1989

Daut RL, Cleeland CS: The prevalence and severity of pain in cancer. Cancer 50:1913–1918, 1982

Davidoff G, Guarracini M, Roth E, et al: Trazodone hydrochloride in the treatment of dysesthetic pain in traumatic myelopathy: a randomized, double-blind, placebo-controlled study. Pain 29:151–161, 1987

Derogatis LR, Morrow GR, Fetting J, et al: The prevalence of psychiatric disorders among cancer patients. JAMA 249:751–757, 1983

Deutschmann W: Tofranil in der Schmerzbehandlung des Krebskranken. Medizinische Welt 22:1346–1347, 1971

Devor M: Nerve pathophysiology and mechanisms of pain in causalgia. J Auton Nerv Syst 7:371–384, 1983

Diamond S, Frietag FG: The use of fluoxetine in the treatment of headache. Clinical Journal of Pain 5:200–201, 1989

Eberhard G, von Knorring L, Nilsson HL, et al: A double-blind randomized study of clomipramine versus maprotiline in patients with idiopathic pain syndromes. Neuropsychobiology 19:25–32, 1988

Farberow NL, Schneidman ES, Leonard CV: Suicide Among General Medical and Surgical Hospital Patients With Malignant Neoplasms, Medical Bulletin 9. Washington DC, U.S. Veterans Administration, 1963

Feighner JP: A comparative trial of fluoxetine and amitriptyline in patients with major depressive disorder. J Clin Psychiatry 46:369–372, 1985

Fernandez F, Adams F, Holmes VF: Analgesic effect of alprazolam in patients with chronic, organic pain of malignant origin. J Clin Psychopharmacol 3:167–169, 1987a

Fernandez F, Adams F, Holmes VF, et al: Methylphenidate for depressive disorders in cancer patients. Psychosomatics 28:455–461, 1987b

Fields HL, Basbaum AI: Endogenous pain control mechanisms, in Textbook of Pain. Edited by Wall PD, Melzak R. London, Churchill Livingston, 1984, pp 142–152

Fiorentino M: Sperimentazione controllata dell' Imipramina come analgesico maggiore in oncologia. Rivista Medica Trentina 5:387–396, 1969

Fishman B, Loscalzo M: Cognitive-behavioral interventions in the management of cancer pain: principles and applications. Med Clin North Am 71:271–287, 1987

Foley KM: Pain syndromes in patients with cancer, in Advances in Pain Research and Therapy, Vol 2. Edited by Bonica JJ, Ventafridda V, Fink RB, et al. New York, Raven, 1975, pp 59–75

Foley KM: The treatment of cancer pain. N Engl J Med 313:84–95, 1985

Forrest WH, Brown Jr BW, Brown CR, et al: Dextroamphetamine with morphine for the treatment of post-operative pain. N Engl J Med 296:712–715, 1977

Fotopoulos SS, Graham C, Cook MR: Psychophysiologic control of cancer pain, in Advances in Pain Research and Therapy. Vol 2. Edited by Bonica JJ, Ventafridda V, Fink RB, et al. New York, Raven, 1979, pp 231–244

France RD: The future for antidepressants: treatment of pain. Psychopathology 20:99–113, 1987

Gebhardt KH, Beller J, Nischk R: Behandlung des Karzinomschmerzes mit Chlorimipramin (Anafranil). Med Klin 64:751–756, 1969

Geller SA: Treatment of fibrositis with fluoxetine hydrochloride (Prozac). Am J Med 87:594–595, 1989

Getto CJ, Sorkness CA, Howell T: Antidepressants and chronic nonmalignant pain: a review. Journal of Pain and Symptom Control 2:9–18, 1987

Gomez-Perez FJ, Rull JA, Dies H, et al: Nortriptyline and fluphenazine in the symptomatic treatment of diabetic neuropathy: a double-blind cross-over study. Pain 23:395–400, 1985

Gram LF: Antidepressants: receptors, pharmacokinetics and clinical effects, in Antidepressants. Edited by Burrows GD, et al. Amsterdam, Elsevier Science, 1983, pp 81–95

Grossman SA, Sheidler VR, Swedeon K, et al: Correlations of patient and caregiver ratings of cancer pain. Journal of Pain and Symptom Management 6:53–57, 1991

Hammeroff SR, Cork RC, Scherer K, et al: Doxepin effects on chronic pain, depression and plasma opioids. J Clin Psychiatry 2:22–26, 1982

Houde RW, Wallenstein SL: Analgesic power of chlorpromazine alone and in combination with morphine (abstract). Fed Proc 14:353, 1966

Hughes A, Chauverghe J, Lissilour T, et al: L'imipramine utilisee comme antalgique majeur en carcinologie: etude de 118 cas. Presse Med 71:1073–1074, 1963

Hynes MD, Lochner MA, Bemis K, et al: Fluoxetine: a selective inhibitor of serotonin uptake, potentiates morphine analgesia without altering its discriminative stimulus properties or affinity for opioid receptors. Life Sci 36:2317–2323, 1985

Kanner RM, Foley KM: Patterns of narcotic use in a cancer pain clinic. Ann N Y Acad Sci 362:161–172, 1981

Katon W, Raskind M: Treatment of depression in the medically ill elderly with methylphenidate. Am J Psychiatry 137:963–965, 1980

Kaufmann MW, Murray GB, Cassem NH: Use of psychostimulants in medically ill depressive patients. Psychosomatics 23:817–819, 1982

King RB: Pain and tryptophan. J Neurosurg 53:44–52, 1980

Kvindesal B, Molin J, Froland A, et al: Imipramine treatment of painful diabetic neuropathy. JAMA 251:1727–1730, 1984

Langohr HD, Stohr M, Petruch F: An open and double-blind crossover study on the efficacy of clomipramine (Anafranil) in patients with painful mono and polyneuropathies. Eur Neurol 21:309–315, 1982

Lascelles RG: Atypical facial pain and depression (letter). Br J Psychol 122:651, 1966

Lechin F, Vander Dijs B, Lechin ME, et al: Pimozide therapy for trigeminal neuralgia. Arch Neurol 9:960–964, 1989

Levin DN, Cleeland CS, Dan R: Public attitudes toward cancer pain. Cancer 56:2337–2339, 1985

Lindblom U, Merskey H, Mumford JM, et al: Pain terms: a current list with definitions and notes on usage. Pain 3:5215, 5221, 1986

Liu SJ, Wang RIH: Increased analgesia and alterations in distribution and metabolism of methadone by desipramine in the rat. J Pharmacol Exp Ther 195:94–104, 1975

Loscalzo M, Jacobsen PB: Practical behavioral approaches to the effective management of pain and distress. Journal of Psychosocial Oncology 8:139–169, 1990

Macaluso C, Weinberg D, Foley KM: Opioid abuse and misuse in a cancer pain population (abstract in Proceedings of the Second Ineternation Congress on Cancer Pain, July 14–17, 1988, Rye, New York). Journal of Pain and Symptom Management 3:54, 1988

Magni G, Arsie D, DeLeo D: Antidepressants in the treatment of cancer pain: a survey in Italy. Pain 29:347–353, 1987

Malseed RT, Goldstein FJ: Enhancement of morphine analgesics by tricyclic antidepressants. Neuropharmacology 18:827–829, 1979

Maltbie AA, Cavenar JO, Sullivan JL, et al: Analgesia and haloperidol: a hypothesis. J Clin Psychiatry 40:323–326, 1979

Marks RM, Sachar EJ: Undertreatment of medical inpatients with narcotic analgesics. Ann Intern Med 78:173–181, 1973

Massie MJ, Holland JC: The cancer patient with pain: psychiatric complications and their management. Med Clin North Am 71:243–258, 1987

Massie JM, Holland JC, Glass E: Delirium in terminally ill cancer patients. Am J Psychiatry 140:1048–1050, 1983

Max MB, Culnane M, Schafer SC, et al: Amitriptyline relieves diabetic-neuropathy pain in patients with normal and depressed mood. Neurology 37:589–596, 1987

Max MB, Schafer SC, Culnane M, et al: Amitriptyline, but not lorazepam, relieves postherpetic neuralgia. Neurology 38:427–432, 1988

Max MB, Kishore-Kumar R, Schafer SC, et al: Efficacy of desipramine in painful diabetic neuropathy: a placebo-controlled trial. Pain 45:3–10, 1991

McKegney FP, Bailey CR, Yates JW: Prediction and management of pain in patients with advanced cancer. Gen Hosp Psychiatry 3:95–101, 1981

Melzack R, Wall PD: The Challenge of Pain. New York, Basic Books, 1983

Merskey H: International Association for the Study of Pain classification of chronic pain: description of chronic pain syndromes and definition of pain terms. Pain 3 (suppl):S1–S225, 1986

Merskey H, Hamilton JT: An open trial of possible analgesic effects of dipyridamole. Journal of Pain Symptom Management 4:34–37, 1989

Monkemeier D, Steffen U: Zur Schmerzbehandlung mit Imipramin bei

Krebserkrankungen. Med Klin 65:213–215, 1970

Munro SM, Mount B: Music therapy in palliative care. Can Med Assoc J 119:1029–1034, 1978

Nehra A, Mullick F, Ishak KG, et al: Pemoline associated hepatic injury. Gastroenterology 99:1517–1519, 1990

Paddison PL, Gise LH, Lebovits A, et al: Sexual abuse and premenstrual syndrome: comparison between a lower and higher socioeconomic group. Psychosomatics 31:265–272, 1990

Passik S, Wilson A: Technical considerations on the frontier of supportive and expressive modes in psychotherapy. Dynamic Psychotherapy 5:51–62, 1987

Pilowsky I, Hallett EC, Bassett DL, et al: A controlled study of amitriptyline in the treatment of chronic pain. Pain 14:169–179, 1982

Portenoy RK, Hagen NA: Breakthrough pain: definition, prevalence and characteristics. Pain 41:273–282, 1990

Redd WB, Reeves JL, Storm FK, et al: Hypnosis in the control of pain during hyperthermia treatment of cancer, in Advances in Pain Research and Therapy, Vol 5. Edited by Bonica JJ, Lindblom U, Iggo A, et al. New York, Raven Press, 1983, pp 857–861

Reik T: Listening With a Third Ear. New York, Farrar, Straus, 1948

Salter MW, Henry JL: Evidence that adenosine moderates the depression of spinal dorsal horn neurones induced by peripheral vibration in the rat. Neuroscience 22:631–650, 1987

Saltzburg D, Breitbart W, Fishman B, et al: The relationship of pain and depression to suicidal ideation in cancer patients (abstract), in Proceedings of the American Society of Clinical Oncology Twenty-Fifth Annual Meeting, May 21–23, 1989, San Francisco, CA. Philadelphia, PA, WB Saunders and American Society of Clinical Oncology, 1989, p 312

Seltzer S, Dewart D, Pollack RL, et al: The effects of dietary tryptophan on chronic maxillofacial pain and experimental pain tolerance. J Psychiatry Res 17:181–186, 1983

Sharav Y, Singer E, Schmidt E, et al: The analgesic effect of amitriptyline on chronic facial pain. Pain 31:199–209, 1987

Silberfarb PM, Manrer LH, Cronthamel CS: Psychological aspects of neoplastic disease, I: functional status of breast cancer patients during different treatment regimens. Am J Psychiatry 137:450–455, 1980

Sindrup SH, Ejlertsen B, Froland A, et al: Imipramine treatment in diabetic neuropathy: relief of subjective symptoms without changes in peripheral and autonomic nerve function. Eur J Clin Pharmacol 37:151–153, 1989

Sindrup SH, Gram LF, Brosen K, et al: The selective serotonin reuptake inhibitor paroxetine is effective in the treatment of diabetic neuropathy symptoms. Pain 42:135–144, 1990

Spiegel D: The use of hypnosis in controlling cancer pain. CA 4:221–231, 1985

Spiegel D, Bloom JR: Pain in metastatic breast cancer. Cancer 52:341–345, 1983a

Spiegel D, Bloom JR: Group therapy and hypnosis reduce metastatic breast carcinoma pain. Psychosom Med 4:333–339, 1983b

Spiegel K, Kalb R, Pasternak GW: Analgesic activity of tricyclic antidepressants. Ann Neurol 13:462-465, 1983

Stiefel FC, Breitbart W, Holland JC: Corticosteroids in cancer: neuropsychiatric complications. Cancer Invest 7:479–491, 1989

Swerdlow M, Cundill JG: Anticonvulsant drugs used in the treatment of lancinating pains: a comparison. Anesthesia 36:1129–1134, 1981

Terr L: Childhood traumas: an outline and overview. Am J Psychiatry 148:10–20, 1991

Theesen KA, Marsh WR: Relief of diabetic neuropathy with fluoxetine. DICP 23:572–574, 1989

Tiegno M, Pagnoni B, Calmi A, et al: Chlorimipramine compared to pentazocine as a unique treatment in postoperative pain. Int J Clin Pharmacol Res 7:141–143, 1987

Turk D, Rennert K: Pain and the terminally ill cancer patient: a cognitive social learning perspective, in Behavior Therapy in Terminal Care: A humanistic Approach. Edited by Sobel H. Cambridge, MA, Ballinger, 1981, 15–44

Twycross RG, Lack SA: Symptom Control in Far Advanced Cancer: Pain Relief. London, Pitman Brooks, 1983

Tyler MA: Treatment of the painful shoulder syndrome with amitriptyline and lithium carbonate. Can Med Assoc J 111:137–140, 1974

Ventafridda V, Bonezzi C, Caraceni A, et al: Antidepressants for cancer pain and other painful syndromes with deafferentation component: comparison of amitriptyline and trazodone. Ital J Neurol Sci 8:579–587, 1987

Ventafridda V, Bianchi M, Ripamonti C, et al: Studies on the effects of antidepressant drugs on the antinociceptive action of morphine and on plasma morphine in rat and man. Pain 43:155–162, 1990

Walker E, Katon W, Griffins JH, et al: Relationship of chronic pelvic pain to psychiatric diagnosis and childhood sexual abuse. Am J Psychiatry 145:75–80, 1988

Walsh TD: Antidepressants and chronic pain. Clin Neuropharmacol 6:271–295, 1983

Walsh TD: Controlled study of imipramine and morphine in chronic pain due to advanced cancer (abstract), in Proceedings of the American Society of Clinical Oncology Twenty-Second Annual Meeting, May 4–6, 1986, Los Angeles, CA. New York, Grune & Stratton and American Society of Clincial Oncology, 1986, p 237

Walsh TD: Adjuvant analgesic therapy in cancer pain, in Advances in Pain

Research and Therapy, Vol 16: Second International Congress on Cancer Pain. Edited by Foley KM, Bonica JJ, Ventafridda V. New York, Raven, 1990, pp 155–165

Watson CP, Evans RJ: A comparative trial of amitriptyline and zimelidine in post-herpetic neuralgia. Pain 23:387–394, 1985

Watson CP, Evans RJ, Reed K, et al: Amitriptyline versus placebo in post herpetic neuralgia. Neurology 32:671–673, 1982

Watson CP, Evans RJ, Reed K, et al: "Therapeutic window" for amitriptyline analgesia (letter). Can Med Assoc J 130:105, 1984

Woodforde JM, Fielding JR: Pain and Cancer. J Psychosom Res 14:365–370, 1970

Young RJ, Clarke BF: Pain relief in diabetic neuropathy: the effectiveness of imipramine and related drugs. Diabetic Med 2:363–366, 1985

Zitman FG, Linssen ACG, Edelbroek PM, et al: Low dose amitriptyline in chronic pain: the gain is modest. Pain 42:35–42, 1990

Chapter 4

Psychiatric Management of Eating Disorders in Cancer Patients

Lynna M. Lesko, M.D., Ph.D.

*C*ancer is notoriously associated with many symptoms of the disease and side effects of its treatment. Common among these symptoms are cachexia and anorexia. *Cachexia* (weight loss) and subsequent failure to gain weight in children and adults with oncological diseases are most often attributed to altered metabolism and negative energy balance (De Wys 1982; Kisner and De Wys 1981). Changes in metabolism in cancer patients are usually manifested in altered carbohydrate and protein metabolism, whereas lipid metabolism is less affected. These metabolic changes usually lead to growth and maturation failure in pediatric patients and muscle wasting in adult patients. Negative energy balance in the cancer patient may be the result of decreased nutritional intake and/or increased nutritional expenditure. Much effort has gone into studying the effects of undernutrition on organ and cell function (Good et al. 1982) and the effect of nutritional status on response to cancer therapy (Van Eys 1982).

Changes in appetite, *anorexia* (loss of appetite), and subsequent weight loss in such patients may result from the malignant disease itself, its treatment (e.g., radiation, surgery, and chemotherapy), concomitant psychological syndromes, preexisting psychiatric syndromes, or behavioral paradigms. In this chapter, the physiological etiology of decreased or insufficient nutritional intake, the psychological mechanisms of cancer anorexia, and various pharmacological, behavioral, and educational interventions currently used are discussed. Other aspects of negative energy balance, increased nutritional expenditure, and altered metabolism are summarized in other excellent review articles (e.g., De Wys 1982).

Pathophysiology of Cancer Cachexia and Anorexia

Cachexia in cancer patients and in the animal model is common but unfortunately complex and not well understood. Anorexia, reduction in caloric intake, and subsequent weight loss have a wide range of central and peripheral causes. As Bernstein (1982) stated, the dilemma is that "the tumor bearing organism fails to increase food intake (and more frequently decreases food intake) in the face of increased energy requirements imposed by tumor growth" (p. S715). In a simplistic model, cachexia in a cancer patient may be the inability to maintain spontaneous food intake in order to keep up with necessary nutritional requirements. Peripheral etiologies of anorexia and cachexia include alterations in sensations of taste and smell, mechanical deficits secondary to surgery, altered physiology caused by radiation and chemotherapy, and primary metabolic effects of tumor growth (inefficient or increased utilization of energy sources). The central regulatory mechanisms of normal food intake, appetite, and cancer anorexia are discussed below.

Anatomically, it is well known from normal animal studies that "lesions" in or "ablation" of the lateral nucleus of the hypothalamus abolishes appetite and causes anorexia, whereas lesions in the ventromedial nucleus result in hyperphagia and weight gain. Unfortunately, lesion-ablation studies in tumor-bearing animals reveal no direct and/or simplistic relationship between anorexia and food intake and hypothalamic region (Bernstein 1982).

Several researchers have also implicated the role of noradrenergic, dopaminergic, serotonergic, and enodorphinergic neurotransmitters in control and modulation of food intake. Elevations in tryptophan and 5-hydroxyindoleacetic acid (5-HIAA: a serotonin metabolite) and depletion of endorphin have been implicated in causing anorexia in tumor-bearing rats (Krause et. al. 1979; Lowry and Yim 1980). Bernstein (1982) added that "the actual role of these transmitters in normal food intake regulation is as yet poorly understood and their role as mediators in cancer anorexia awaits further research" (p. S715).

Cancer-related cachexia may be explained by accelerated losses in skeletal protein. Some investigators feel that the rate of protein loss is greater in fed tumor-bearing animals than in fed control animals (Norton et al. 1981) and suggest that there is a "tumor-induced" acceleration of skeletal protein loss independent of food intake. More recently, cachectin or tumor necrosis factor (TNF), a protein secreted by macrophages (which is disseminated via the circulation to interact with receptors on various end organs), has been implicated as an important central mediator in inducing toxic shock and wasting (cachexia) in animal models (Beutler 1988; Beutler and Cerami 1987; Olds 1985). Cachectin produces a picture of weight loss, poor food intake, and apathy, as well as fever in animals. Elucidation of this important protein's mode of action may enhance our understanding of this problem in cancer.

Physiological Causes of Anorexia-Cachexia Syndrome Secondary to Cancer and Its Treatment

The anorexia-cachexia syndrome in patients with oncological disease has physiological and psychological causes. Table 4–1 includes a comprehensive list of the physiological (i.e., disease- and treatment-related) causes of cancer anorexia. The psychological aspects of cancer anorexia (e.g., depression, psychological distress, and behavioral paradigms such as learned food aversions) are discussed below. (For a concise background on the physiological causes of cancer anorexia, see review articles by Holland et al. 1977, Ohnuma and Holland 1977, and Shils 1979, as well as the more recent volume edited by Burish et al. 1985.)

Disease-Related Anorexia

Anorexia and secondary weight loss can occur early in the course of certain gastrointestinal (GI) cancers such as those of the stomach, colon, rectum, and pancreas and in some cases can be the sole presenting symptom. Occasionally, these symptoms are misinterpreted as depressive symptomatology, and the patient is mistakenly referred to a psychiatrist. Metabolic abnormalities such as fever, anemia, uremia, hepatic dysfunction, protein-losing enteropathy, and other malabsorption difficulties can all produce transient anorexia in a patient at various stages of a malignant illness. These abnormalities may disrupt the feeding-satiety center of the hypothalamus, producing decreased hunger or early satiety. A growing area of interest concerning nutritional problems in lung cancer is the secretion of ectopic hormones, kinins,

Table 4–1.   Physiological causes of eating disorders in cancer patients

Disease related
    Cancer cachexia syndrome
    Early symptoms of pancreatic or gastrointestinal cancer
    Tumor obstruction by advancing disease
    Fever
    Chronic illness, anemia
    Metabolic (uremia and hepatic dysfunction)
    Protein-losing enteropathy (gastric cancer)
    Ectopic hormone production by tumors (lung)
    Pain or discomfort

Treatment related
    Surgery
        Oropharyngeal resection: loss of dentition, chewing and swallowing
            difficulties
        Esophagectomy and reconstruction: gastric acid secondary to
            vagotomy, fibrosis
        Gastrectomy: gastric acid, malabsorption, "dumping" syndrome
        Pancreatectomy: diabetes, malabsorption
        Bowel resection: malabsorption, diarrhea secondary to bile salt
            loss, malnutrition
        Ileostomy or colostomy: fluid electrolyte imbalance
    Drug related
        Chemotherapeutic agents: fluid and electrolyte imbalance
            secondary to nausea and vomiting, stomatitis of alimentary canal,
        abdominal pain, constipation, intestinal ulceration, diarrhea,
            neuropathy, central nervous system complications
        Pain medication: somnolence, constipation
        Antifungal and antibacterial agents
    Radiation therapy
        Oropharyngeal area: taste and smell, stomatitis
        Neck and mediastinal area: dysphagia, esophagitis, esophageal
            fibrosis stenosis, fistulas
        Abdomen-pelvic area: nausea, vomiting, diarrhea, malabsorption,
            stenosis, fistulas
    Other
        Graft-versus-host disease (bone marrow transplantation): diarrhea,
            electrolyte imbalance, malabsorption

Source.   Adapted from Lesko L: "Anorexia," in *Handbook of Psychooncology:
Psychological Care of the Patient With Cancer.* Edited by Holland JC, Rowland
JH. New York, Oxford University Press, 1989, pp. 434–443.

and various polypeptides. Such agents may affect peripheral or central systems to produce decreased appetite. Finally, pain, discomfort, and GI obstruction can all lead to transient but profound anorexia in the later stages of disease.

Treatment-Related Anorexia

Anorexia can be a pervasive symptom secondary to a patient's cancer treatment. Loss of appetite can be caused by surgery, radiation, and/or chemotherapy (Table 4–1). Many of the chemotherapeutic drugs alone or in combination with radiation may produce anorexia secondary to their effects on the hypothalamus or by their emetic potential.

The effects of ablative surgery for cancer on taste and nutrition can often be profound, complicating the later chemotherapy- and radiation-induced anorexia. Ablative radical head and neck surgery can result in loss of normal oral architecture and/or decreased function (masticating and swallowing). The taste of food and pleasure of eating can be altered by extensive upper-GI surgery. Such surgery may require prolonged feedings via a nasogastric tube. Such indwelling tubes can produce throat irritation and psychological trauma that interferes with appetite and the quality and sensation of taste and food intake. Gastrectomy and bowel resection can result in malabsorption and weight loss. Temporary or permanent colostomy in a small number of patients produces psychological trauma centered around food intake and excretion. Secondary anorexia and decreased oral intake can ensue. Pancreatic resection and resultant lost of endocrine function can produce alterations in insulin control and subsequent nausea and decreased appetite.

Radiation therapy can cause transient and permanent sequelae that interfere with taste and oral consumption of nutrients. Radiation-induced anorexia often depends on the amount of radiation, the length of radiation treatments, and the targeted area of such treatment. Immediate effects of radiation treatment can often produce stomatitis, mucositis pharyngitis, esophagitis, nausea and/or vomiting, and diarrhea. Permanent and often more serious sequelae affecting appetite can develop. These involve a decreased sense of or change in taste (Huldij et al. 1986), change in saliva production, dysphagia secondary to esophageal fibrosis, and lower-GI obstruction secondary to stenosis or fistualization. Any time the oral canal, the senses involved in eating (i.e., smell and taste), or the secondary organ systems (i.e., saliva production) are affected by treatment, the experience of food intake is limited and anorexia may develop.

Nausea, vomiting, decreased oral intake, fluid and electrolyte imbalance, and subsequent anorexia can be produced by almost all chemotherapeutic agents (e.g., cyclophosphamide [Cytoxan], nitrogen mustards, and cisplatin). Only a few agents, such as the alkylating agents (vincristine) and corticosteroids, are not associated with nausea, vomiting, and subsequent anorexia. Chemotherapy agents such as vincristine can, however, produce constipation and ileus resulting in anorexia. Stomatitis with oral ulcerations, glossitis, pharyngitis, and esophagitis are extremely common with methotrexate, fluorouracil, and high-dose doxorubicin (Adriamycin). Due to the rapid turnover of epithelial cells of the mucosal layer of the alimentary canal, the GI tract is extremely vulnerable to side effects of these agents resulting in ulcerations, pain, and anorexia. Drugs other than chemotherapy agents (e.g., antibiotics and antifungal and pain medications) can produce transient anorexic syndromes. Analgesics may produce central nervous system somnolence, resulting in missed meals and poor nutrition.

A very serious long-term consequence of high-dose chemotherapy, radiation, and bone marrow transplantation is graft-versus-host disease (GVHD). Despite matching of donor and recipient at the major histocompatible antigen sites and adequate postgraft immunosuppression, 70% of patients can develop a GVHD syndrome (Deeg and Storb 1986). Principal target organs of this syndrome include skin, GI tract, and liver. GI dysfunction, usually manifest after the typical skin rash, is characterized by diarrhea, abdominal pain, ileus, anorexia, weight loss, malabsorption, and failure to thrive. Newer treatments of donor bone marrow with lectins and monoclonal antibodies can in most cases virtually do away with GVHD and its sequelae.

Psychological Aspects of Cancer Anorexia

Even though anorexia is one of the most common symptoms of malignancy, it is the most difficult to treat due to its multiple etiologies. We often overlook the psychological causes and dynamics of anorexia in our haste to intervene (Table 4–2). In this section, loss of appetite is discussed in the context of psychiatric syndromes, learned food aversions, and behavioral issues. Case examples are included to illustrate the often complex nature of anorexia.

Psychiatric Causes of Appetite Loss

Often anorexia in patients with malignancies is seen in the context of an anxiety syndrome. We mistakenly make light of the complaint "I just don't feel like eating" and chalk it up to side effects of treatment or disease. It is well known in psychiatric literature that patients without medical illness, but with symptoms of anxiety or depression, can expe-

Table 4–2.   Psychological causes of eating disorders in cancer patients

Anxiety
   Fears related to meaning of weight loss, assumed to be associated with tumor progression
   Concerns about inability to eat
   Issues about loss of normal appetite

Depression
   Loss of appetite
   Weight loss
   Dysphoria
   Hopelessness, helplessness
   Withdrawal

Delirium
   Altered mental status secondary to disease and its treatment

Psychiatric disorders
   Anorexia nervosa
   Affective disorders
   Schizophrenic disorders
   Personality disorders
   Paranoia (suspiciousness of poisoning and refusal to eat)

Food aversions
   Specific food aversions: decreased protein tolerance, increased glucose tolerance
   Learned food aversions

Behavioral
   Anticipatory nausea and vomiting

Source.   Adapted from Lesko L: "Anorexia," in *Handbook of Psychooncology: Psychological Care of the Patient With Cancer.* Edited by Holland JC, Rowland JH. New York, Oxford University Press, 1989, pp. 434–443.

rience a decreased interest in appetite and food intake. At the time of a cancer diagnosis, appetite is exquisitely sensitive to anxious mood. On learning the diagnosis of cancer, many patients note that, along with signs of distress such as insomnia and poor concentration, they lose their appetite. The loss of a few pounds is enough to frighten such patients even more; their first assumption is that the recently diagnosed cancer is causing the weight loss. Reassurance about the emotional turmoil they are feeling may have an impact on appetite and is often enough to reduce the anxiety and encourage a return to normal food intake. Occasionally, benzodiazepines are necessary to control levels of anxiety. The fear of relapse and recurrence is greatest immediately after ending treatment, but it does not ever fully disappear. Concerned and anxious family members, alarmed by signs of poor eating, may attempt to force food on cancer patients, making eating the source of family conflict. In some individuals, the fear of weight loss and its potential significance as a sign of tumor progression leads to compulsive overeating. This is of equal concern; forced eating in the absence of hunger, as a compulsive habit, can result in obesity and appears most often in women with breast cancer undergoing chemotherapy. The following case example illustrates the alarm that can be generated in patients and their families when eating difficulties and weight loss complicate surgery for a cancer of the gastrointestinal tract:

Case 1

Mr. L, a 63-year-old widower, had a gastrectomy for an early gastric carcinoma. He was previously anxious and had a history of several phobias. His postoperative course was complicated by anxiety attacks, chronic fears, and difficulty in eating and maintaining weight. Mr. L and his family were convinced that the problems with eating were due to recurrence of cancer. A psychiatric consultation was requested to help him deal with anxiety; however, it soon became clear that some of his difficulty in eating was also related to uncontrolled anxiety. Intervention included psychotherapy, medication (antianxiety drugs), and repeated visits to the surgeon to reassure Mr. L and his daughter that the symptoms were not physical in origin, but rather an exacerbation of a previous psychiatric condition.

Anorexia can be a cardinal symptom of depression, but it is also a major symptom of advanced cancer. It is in the advanced stages where both are more common and the differential diagnosis between major depression and physical origin of anorexia becomes a difficult problem. Anorexia may be a consequence of the medical situation that results in secondary depression and further inability to eat, or depression may be the prime contributor to anorexia. Patients may begin to feel helpless in the face of continuing anorexia and weight loss leading to despair and hopelessness. Such painful emotional states require intervention. It is important to make an accurate assessment of possible physical and psychological contributors to anorexia. Treatment of the psychological component includes counseling and pharmacological interventions aimed directly at appetite and at depressive symptoms. Often a therapeutic trial of an antidepressant medication is worth attempting even when a diagnosis of major depression is not firm. The following case example illustrates how major psychiatric and intra-abdominal pathology can interact:

Case 2

Ms. M, a 61-year-old woman with pancreatic cancer, was treated with chemotherapy but experienced profound anorexia, weight loss, and abdominal pain. Subsequently, she developed severe depression and withdrawal, which her psychiatrist felt were due to a combination of functional (anticipatory mourning) and organic (pain medicines) factors. She wished to be treated at her daughter's home and was kept comfortable by family and home care nursing. Her treatment regimen included analgesics, antidepressants (those with minimal sedating effects), and low-dose amphetamine. Frequent psychotherapeutic home visits with her husband and children during the 3 months in which the disease progressed were useful in symptom control of depression, anorexia, and overall family anxiety.

Preexisting psychiatric disorders in individuals who develop cancer can complicate their care and contribute to anorexia. In particular, affective and schizophrenic syndromes, personality disorders, and anorexia nervosa can result in altered intake and weight loss. Patients with such disorders present very complicated treatment issues. Anorexia nervosa, common among young women, has constituted a particularly difficult problem in anorexic individuals who are later treated with chemotherapy (with its concomitant nausea and vomiting). Weight loss, unusual difficulty with taste, and relentless preoccupation with food may not be related to the physical illness, but evidence of a concurrent and complicating psychiatric disorder, as the following case example illustrates:

Case 3

Ms. N was diagnosed at age 21 as having acute leukemia. The fifth of seven children, she had come to the United States with her parents from Greece. Her leukemia treatment was uneventful until, during a second relapse, she began to "fake" taking drugs at home to avoid the nausea and vomiting, even injecting saline to fool her family. After the second relapse, she was hospitalized for an allogenic bone marrow transplantation. Her hospital course was complicated by a longer-than-normal weaning period from total parenteral nutrition and disinterest in follow-up. Over 3 years, she had anorexia, had difficulty swallowing, was unable to take food except iced tea, and did not take oral medications regularly at home.

Ms. N was evaluated by several psychiatrists who felt she had had early symptoms of anorexia nervosa (before leukemia), which were exacerbated by the transplantation procedure. She was hospitalized for infections, dehydration, failure to thrive, and weight loss. Her complaints of anorexia and difficulty swallowing continued; finally she refused to eat because it would "make me feel ugly." Her family, who were immigrants and could barely speak English, focused their attention on her cachexia, interpreting the symptoms as due to the leukemia. Ms. N's noncompliance and passivity in the face of efforts to maintain her oral intake necessitated placement of a percutaneous feeding tube. She complained of bloating, abdominal pain, and diarrhea. Eventually she became immunologically compromised and died of generalized sepsis and failure to thrive.

Learned Food Aversions

Recently it has been suggested that appetite suppression in some cancer patients may be due to "learned food aversions" (Bernstein 1978, 1982, 1986; Bernstein and Sigundi 1980; Bernstein and Webster 1985; Bernstein et al. 1979; Mattes et al. 1987). According to Bernstein and colleagues (see Bernstein and Webster 1985), who use animal models to study cancer anorexia, learned food aversions are acquired to specific foods or tastes which develop as a result of the association of these foods with unpleasant internal symptoms (i.e., nausea and vomiting).

This behavioral phenomenon of conditioned or learned taste aversion is similar to classical conditioning paradigms in which animals learn to associate a conditioned stimulus (taste) with an unconditioned response (symptom of the illness). In animal models, 1) it is possible to introduce a delay of many hours between the conditioned stimulus and the subsequent discomfort (unconditioned response), and 2) the acquisition of such learning can occur rapidly with only one trial.

In an attempt to examine this response in humans, Bernstein (1978) examined learned food aversions in children receiving chemotherapy for cancer. These elegant studies are of particular importance because this phenomenon had not been previously demonstrated in humans. Children receiving chemotherapy (producing moderate to severe nausea and vomiting) were randomized to control or experimental groups. Patients in the experimental group were offered a novel food (maple toffee ice cream) shortly before their scheduled chemotherapy treatment. Patients in one control group received no novel food but were occupied with a toy. Other control groups consisted of patients receiving chemotherapy with little emetic potency or patients receiving no chemotherapy at all. All patients were tested for food aversions to the ice cream at 1 to 4 weeks. Patients exposed to the novel food stimulus were three times more likely to develop a significant food aversion than patients in the control groups ($P<.01$). These studies were expanded to determine whether patients receiving chemotherapy regimens developed food aversions to common, preferred, or familiar foods. The researchers concluded that food aversions are fairly specific to food eaten before therapy that produces GI distress, and they may occur not only with novel foods presented before chemotherapy but also with regular foods in the patient's diet, which may have been eaten up to several hours before treatment. Other studies by Bernstein and colleagues (see Bernstein and Sigundi 1980) in animal models have indicated that learned food aversions can occur in animals that are anorexic secondary to tumor growth. However, they demonstrated that it was possible to increase caloric intake by presenting a novel diet.

In summary, both clinical and laboratory studies have indicated that learned food aversions in cancer patients result from both treatment and tumor growth and suggest an interesting but causal role in the development of tumor anorexia. Such a food aversion model has been used to test various interventions for eliminating or reducing such problems. In these studies (e.g., Broberg and Bernstein 1987) the only intervention that significantly lowered the magnitude of drug-induced food aversion was the presentation of a novel food or diet on the days of treatment. These preliminary studies using animal models are useful in identifying potential interventions effective in clinical practice.

Occasionally, eating itself may result in biochemical changes and altered metabolism, which in turn may precipitate a learned food aversion. De Wys (1982) noted that patients with cancer produce elevated levels of lactate, a metabolite known to cause nausea if infused into control subjects. De Wys suggested that cancer patients eating even a normal-size meal or a high-carbohydrate diet may develop nausea, which then in turn becomes a learned response.

This final case example presents the interplay between the psychological (anxiety and conflict around weaning from total parenteral nutrition and subsequent discharge), physiological (liver damage and change in taste secondary to radiation and chemotherapy), and behavioral (learned food aversions) etiologies of anorexia. The psychological intervention for this patient was multimodal and included behavioral and pharmacological management. The patient's liver dysfunction slowly resolved without any physiological treatment.

Case 4

Mr. O, a 51-year-old man with acute leukemia, was treated with a chemotherapy regimen of induction and consolidation that resulted in acute but transient episodes of nausea, vomiting, anorexia, and change in taste. He was then rapidly admitted to a sterile room for an allogenic bone marrow transplantation. Over 3 months he received hyperalimentation, which was necessary secondary to stomatitis. Weaning from parenteral nutrition was stormy; despite absence of any physical problem, he had severe anorexia. However, after struggles with his physician who wanted him to eat more, he was discharged with continued anorexia and nausea. After a week at home on a bland diet, Mr. O became dehydrated and was started on parenteral nutrition. He became depressed and developed nausea first to solids and then to semisolids. Finally the smell of food or sight of his menu resulted in anxiety and nausea. Antiemetics in adequate doses produced side effects, and he was finally successfully treated by desensitization and relaxation.

Clinical Management of Anorexia and Eating Disorders

Although cancer anorexia may for the most part be physiological and metabolic in nature, psychological interventions may be extremely useful in its treatment. Current and promising interventions such as psychopharmacological agents and psychoeducational-behavioral techniques are highlighted below.

In caring for the patient with cancer-related anorexia, a full assessment of the physiological causes of altered metabolism, appetite change, and decreased food intake metabolism is required. The reassurance gained by a patient from an understanding of the cause of the anorexia is critically important. Involving both the patient and family members is critical. Weekly supportive sessions will often begin with a review of appetite changes as a sign of progress toward feeling better. Assessment and treatment of underlying anxiety or depression or potential personal problems contributing to anorexia must be part of each evaluation. Referral for diet education or behavioral interventions is always helpful and often critical for patient management. Books and information on high-caloric foods, how to serve tasteful meals, new recipes, and other techniques for increasing food intake, such as frequent meals, are useful.

Pharmacological Intervention

Several pharmacological agents are known to be useful in promoting weight gain in patients with oncological disease (Holland et al. 1977). They include antihistamines (cyproheptadine), steroids (dexamethasone and prednisone), amphetamine-like agents (dexamphetamine and methylphenidate), antidepressants with anticholinergic effects (tricyclic antidepressants), cannabinoids (tetrahydrocannabinols [Δ^9-THC]), and progestational agents (megestrol) (Table 4–3).

It is often difficult to separate out whether appetite loss in cancer patients is due to the tumor or cancer therapy or represents an early symptom of depression. As mentioned above, appetite loss may be the first symptom of depression in cancer patients. In particular, elderly patients may exhibit only one or two of the cardinal symptoms of depression, which include weight loss, anorexia, or difficulty sleeping. Consequently, a trial of an antidepressant (in low doses) can be extremely helpful to patients in regaining their appropriate food intake. Steroids can produce a mild euphoria and an enhanced sense of well-being that initially improves appetite. Over time, however, increased appetite can result in obesity and severe problems in controlling weight.

Megestrol acetate, used in breast cancer regimens, may promote increased appetite and subsequent weight gain and may prove an important pharmacological intervention for anorexia and cachexia in terminal illness and acquired immunodeficiency syndrome (AIDS) (Loprinzi et al. 1990; Tchekmedyian et al. 1986, 1992; Von Roenn et al. 1988). Cruz et al. (1990) studied approximately 200 women with advanced breast cancer, comparing a standard regimen of 160 mg per day with one of 800 mg per day; weight gain was directly correlated to the dose and length of megestrol acetate treatment. Megestrol acetate, at a dose of 160 mg per day, resulted in a 5-lb weight gain in a significant portion of cancer patients (none with breast cancer)

Table 4–3. Pharmacological interventions in the management of cancer-related eating disorders

Pharmacological drug (trade name)	Class	Dose
Cyproheptadine (Periactin)	Antihistamine	4 mg po tid (tablet or elixir)
Dexamethasone (Decadron); prednisone	Steroids	Variable
Dextroamphetamine (Dexedrine)	Amphetamine[a]	5–10 mg bid
Methylphenidate (Ritalin)	Stimulant	2.5–5 mg bid
Tricyclic antidepressants	Antidepressant	25–100 mg/day
Tetrahydrocannabinols [Δ^9-THC]	Cannabinoids	15 mg/day po or inhalation
Megestrol acetate (Megace)	Progestational	160–800 mg/day
Hydrazine sulfate		60 mg po tid

[a]Should be taken in morning or early afternoon to prevent insomnia.
Source.   Adapted from Lesko L: "Anorexia," in *Handbook of Psychooncology: Psychological Care of the Patient With Cancer.* Edited by Holland JC, Rowland JH. New York, Oxford University Press, 1989, pp. 434–443.

(Tchekmedyian et al. 1986). In a large randomized, double-blind, placebo-controlled trial (Loprinzi et al. 1990) of megestrol acetate in patients with cancer-associated anorexia and cachexia, patients receiving 800 mg per day of megestrol experienced significant appetite stimulation and weight gain (16% gained 15 lb or more) with little associated toxicity. Tchekmedyian et al. (1987) have also studied high-dose regimens of megestrol acetate (e.g., 480–1600 mg per day) and found that such a regimen could be helpful in cancer anorexia. The experience with doses of megestrol acetate in excess of 800 mg per day is limited, however, and care should be exercised with any use of this drug above such a dose (Bruera 1992).

Amphetamine and amphetamine-like agents also stimulate appetite. Small doses of dextroamphetamine or methylphenidate in the morning reduce the withdrawal and apathy experienced by patients with advanced disease and also reduce somnolence caused by analgesics. Excessive doses, however, reduce appetite and if given toward evening can inhibit sleep. Dizziness, somnolence, depersonalization, and dysphoria can occur with cannabinoids at doses sufficient to improve appetite, thereby limiting their usefulness.

Hydrazine sulfate is a drug currently under study as a potentially useful agent in the treatment of cancer anorexia and cachexia. In a study (Chleboweki et al. 1987) of 101 patients, 83% maintained or increased their weight on hydrazine sulfate 60 mg tid, compared to 58% in the placebo group. Further studies of hydrazine sulfate are planned.

Behavioral and Educational Techniques

Quite often, simple behavioral and educational techniques are overlooked by distraught patients and their families. Some very basic behavioral techniques can be used by hospital staff and families to improve oral intake and possibly reverse symptoms of appetite loss (Table 4–4). A dietary consultation can be helpful in educating patients and families on the nutritional content of certain foods, especially those high in calories and protein; the necessity for small and frequent meals; novel ways of preparing favorite foods; and new recipes with tempting visual presentations. Often such a consultation is mandatory when a patient has undergone head and neck surgery and requires special pureed foods or prosthetic devices. Patients receiving chemotherapy or radiation often avoid strongly flavored foods like barbecued meats or fish and may prefer canned fruits, cottage cheese, or milk supplements. Stomatitis secondary to radiation or chemotherapy and oral candidal infections involve not only the oral mucosa, but also the esophagus, and patients with such conditions may require pureed or liquid foods because of pain.

Radiation and mucosal GVHD may change the characteristics of the patient's saliva or decrease it's volume, necessitating more liquid with meals or saliva-like additives to moisten the oral cavity. In these situations, saliva becomes "thick and difficult to cough up"; patients do not tolerate milk products that appear to aggravate this problem. In addition, candidal infections treated with oral medications (nystatin) often make food taste undesirable. If anorexia and decreased caloric intake become profound, nutritional consultation may be necessary for artificial feeding, either "enteral" through a nasogastric tube or feeding gastrostomy, or "parenteral" via a Hickman-Broviac catheter.

The ambiance at meal time can be very important for improving caloric intake. Having a family member share a meal with the hospitalized patient, serving a favorite wine or beer, or using candles and special table settings can add many of the social aspects that physically well individuals associate with a pleasant meal. If possible, a gathering of two or three patients who can eat communally creates an ambiance more conducive to joyful and pleasurable eating.

Table 4–4. Psychoeducational-supportive and behavioral interventions in the management of cancer-related eating disorders

---

Psychoeducational-supportive

Supportive psychotherapy for fears and psychiatric issues related to weight loss

Advice about meals with high caloric and protein content, appetizing recipes, visually appealing presentations, creating an ambiance at mealtime, novel ways of preparing favorite foods

Special consultation for medically related problems of head and neck tumors, stomatitis, artificial feeding

Behavioral

Relaxation techniques to reduce anxiety and anticipatory phenomena before meals

Techniques to reduce learned food aversions

Operant conditioning methods for weight gain

A variety of more sophisticated behavioral techniques have been applied to eating disorders in cancer, especially among children. Because anorexia may be accompanied by anxiety, worry concerning food intake, and anticipatory anxiety or nausea before a meal, the fear, anxiety, worry, and anorexia may become behaviorally linked to one another. In such situations, several behavioral techniques, such as relaxation or self-hypnosis, can lower anxiety and anticipatory phenomena around eating and improve fluid and caloric intake. Conflicts about eating often necessitate meetings with staff and family members. Attention to situations that create problems and are associated with refusal to eat are important and should be recognized early in the course of the illness. If anxiety is the center of the problem, relaxation exercises before meals in an effort to reduce the focus on eating and diminish anticipatory distress symptoms coupled with use of anxiolytic medication can improve the anorexia. Sometimes patients complain of nausea at the thought or sight of food, and relaxation with an antiemetic may be appropriate. Symptoms may be experienced more in socially embarrassing situations, such as in a restaurant, in which the inability to eat or nausea increases patients' self-consciousness and may become a reason to remain at home and not eat with others.

Contingency management, in which rewards such as family visits, exercise, watching television, or tokens are dependent on weight gain or caloric intake, have been successful in patients with primary anorexia nervosa. There has been no research in the literature to say whether this behavioral method can be applied to cancer patients with anorexia. However, a few cancer patients may develop secondary anorexia nervosa, indistinguishable from that seen in the psychiatric population. The etiology of this syndrome is unknown; one theory is that anorexic-like features or characteristics that had been dormant in some individuals were triggered by the cancer diagnosis and its treatment. An operant conditioning-based treatment may be of help in such patients (W. H. Redd, personal communication, June 1989).

Summary

Cancer anorexia with its associated decreased food intake and weight loss is a common and profoundly important symptom in malignancy, and one that has at times a psychological as well as a physical component. Most poorly understood is the anorexia-cachexia syndrome of advanced disease. When physical in origin, it may be caused directly or indirectly by the disease process or treatment. Psychological causes often reflect anxiety about cancer, its possible progression, depression, anticipatory phenomena, and learned food aversions. Preexisting psychiatric disorders, especially anorexia nervosa or paranoid states, can substantially complicate cancer treatment. Recent research indicates that learned food aversions may play a role in cancer anorexia and can occur as a result of the pairing or association of foods with tumor growth or with the side effects of chemotherapy.

The management of nutrition in the oncological setting can be enhanced by the use of various types of artificial feeding (i.e., parenteral or enteral administration) and by judicious use of various pharmacological drugs that control nausea and vomiting or stimulate appetite. Regardless of etiology, psychological management of the anorexia is often helpful. Optimal management often involves the use of a combination of modalities: psychotherapeutic, behavioral, and/or pharmacological supplemented by education, counseling, and support. Behavioral techniques such as relaxation exercises are useful tools to alter this response as well as to relieve the anxiety precipitated by patient concerns about anorexia and weight loss. Environmental interventions and nutritional advice can also be of considerable value in reversing the negative effects of this distressing symptom in cancer. Artificial feeding, used for poor intake (Brennan 1981), poses a special set of psychological problems for patient and family depending on whether it is accomplished by tubes (enteral) or catheters (parenteral) (Lesko 1989).

References

Bernstein IL: Learned taste aversion in children receiving chemotherapy. Science 200:1302–1303, 1978

Bernstein IL: Physiological and psychological mechanisms of cancer anorexia. Cancer Res 42 (suppl):S715–S720, 1982

Bernstein IL: Etiology of anorexia in cancer. Cancer 581:1881–1886, 1986

Bernstein IL, Sigundi RA: Tumor anorexia: a learned food aversion. Science 209:416–418, 1980

Bernstein IL, Webster MM: Learned food aversions: a consequence of cancer chemotherapy, in Cancer, Nutrition and Eating Behavior. Edited by Burish TG, Levy SM, Meyerowitz BE. Hillsdale, NJ, Lawrence Earlbaum, 1985, pp 103–116

Bernstein IL, Wallace MI, Bernstein ID, et al: Learned food aversions as a consequence of cancer treatment, in Nutrition and Cancer. Edited by Van Eys J, Seelig MS, Nichols BL. New York, SP Medical & Scientific Books, 1979, pp 159–164

Beutler B: Cachexia: a fundamental mechanism. Nutr Rev 46:369–373, 1988

Beutler B, Cerami T: Cachectin: more than a tumor necrosis factor. N Engl J Med 316:379–385, 1987

Brennan MF: Total parenteral nutrition in the cancer patient. N Engl J Med 305:375–381, 1981

Broberg DJ, Bernstein IL: Candy as a scapegoat in the prevention of food aversions in children receiving chemotherapy. Cancer 60:2344–2347, 1987

Bruera E: Current pharmacological management of anorexia in cancer patients. Oncology 6:125–137, 1992

Burish TG, Levy SM, Meyerowitz BE: Cancer, Nutrition and Eating Behavior. Hillsdale, NJ, Lawrence Earlbaum, 1985

Chlebowski RT, Bulcavage L, Grosvenor M, et al: Hydrazine sulfate in cancer patients with weight loss: a placebo-controlled clinical experience. Cancer 59:406–410, 1987

Cruz JM, Mus HB, Brockschmidt JK, et al: Weight changes in women with metastatic breast cancer treated with megestrol acetate: a comparison of standard versus high dose therapy. Seminars in Oncology 17 (suppl 9):S63–S67, 1990

Deeg HJ, Storb R: Acute and chronic graft versus host disease. J Natl Cancer Inst 76(6):1325–1328, 1986

De Wys WD: Pathophysiology of cancer cachexia: current understanding and areas for future research. Cancer Res 42 (suppl):721S–726S, 1982

Good RA, West A, Day NK, et al: Effects of undernutrition on host cell and organ function. Cancer Res 42 (suppl):737S–746S, 1982

Holland JC, Rowland JH, Plumb M: Psychological aspects of anorexia in cancer patients. Cancer Res 37:2425–2428, 1977

Huldij A, Giesberg A, Klein Poelhuis EH, et al: Alterations in taste appreciation in cancer patients during treatment. Cancer Nurs 9:38–42, 1986

Kisner DL, De Wys WD: Anorexia and cachexia in malignant disease, in Nutrition and Cancer: Etiology and Treatment. Edited by Newell GR, Ellison NM. New York, Raven, 1981, pp 355–365

Krause R, James JH, Ziparo V, et al: Brain tryptophan and the neoplastic anorexia-cachexia syndrome. Cancer 44:1003–1008, 1979

Lesko L: Anorexia, in Handbook of Psychooncology: Psychological Care of the Patient With Cancer. Edited by Holland JC, Rowland JH. New York, Oxford University Press, 1989, pp 434–443

Loprinzi CL, Ellison NM, Schaid DJ, et al: Controlled trial of megestrol acetate for the treatment of cancer anorexia and cachexia. J Natl Cancer Inst 82:1127–1132, 1990

Lowry MT, Yim GKW: Similar feeding profiles in tumor-bearing and dexamethasone-treated rats suggest endorphin depletion in cancer cachexia. Neuroscience Abstracts 6:518, 1980

Mattes RD, Arnold C, Borass M: Learned food aversions among cancer chemotherapy patients: incidence, nature and clinical implications. Cancer 60:2576–2580, 1987

Norton JA, Shamberger R, Stein TP, et al: The influence of tumor-bearing on protein metabolism in the rat. J Surg Res 30:456–462, 1981

Ohnuma T, Holland JF: Nutritional consequences of cancer chemotherapy and immunotherapy. Cancer Res 37:2395–2406, 1977

Olds LJ: Tumor necrosis factor (TNF). Science 230:630–632, 1985

Shils ME: Nutritional problems induced by cancer. Med Clin North Am 63:1009–1025, 1979

Tchekmedyian NS, Tait N, Moody M, et al: Appetite stimulation with megestrol acetate in cachectic cancer patients. Semin Oncol 13:37–43, 1986

Tchekmedyian NS Tait N, Moody M, et al: High dose megestrol acetate: a possible treatment for cachexia. JAMA 257:1195–1199, 1987

Tchekmedyian NS, Hickman M, Sian J, et al: Megestrol acetate in cancer anorexia and weight loss. Cancer 69:1268–1274, 1992

Van Eys J: Effects of nutritional status on response to therapy. Cancer Res 42 (suppl):747S–753S, 1982

Von Roenn JH, Murphy RL, Weber KM, et al: Megestrol acetate for treatment of cachexia associated with human immunodeficiency virus (HIV) infection. Ann Intern Med 109:840–849, 1988

Chapter 5

Anticipatory Nausea and Vomiting With Cancer Chemotherapy

Michael A. Andrykowski, Ph.D.
Paul B. Jacobsen, Ph.D.

*M*any cancer patients experience nausea and vomiting after infusions of chemotherapeutic agents. This posttreatment nausea and vomiting (PNV) is presumed to be pharmacological in origin although the contribution of psychological and physiological factors is increasingly being recognized (Jacobsen et al. 1988). In addition, some patients become nauseated or experience episodes of vomiting before receiving a chemotherapy infusion. Typically, such anticipatory nausea and vomiting (ANV) is triggered by in vivo exposure to certain stimuli associated with the administration of chemotherapy; for example, a characteristic hospital or clinic odor or the sight of the clinic waiting room or treatment area may elicit nausea and vomiting. In some cases, even the thought of receiving chemotherapy is sufficient to trigger nausea and vomiting. Because these symptoms appear in the absence of any pharmacological stimulus, ANV is presumed to be primarily psychological rather than pharmacological in origin.

ANV has been the focus of numerous clinical and empirical reports (Burish and Carey 1986; Carey and Burish 1988; Morrow and Dobkin 1988; Redd and Andrykowski 1982). Interest in ANV has been stimulated by its status as both a clinically and theoretically significant phenomenon. Clinically, ANV is both physically and emotionally stressful for patients and can influence their decision to discontinue chemotherapy (Weddington 1982). Moreover, patients, friends, and family members often believe that these symptoms reflect psychopathology or psychological weakness, a misperception that is unfortunately shared by some health professionals (Chang 1981) and may actually serve to further patients' distress. Theoretically, ANV presents a rare opportunity to study the natural process of aversion learning in humans. An understanding of the basic processes involved in ANV development can then guide clinical efforts toward prevention and treatment of these symptoms.

In this chapter, we discuss four issues concerning the phenomenon of ANV: 1) the prevalence of ANV, 2) factors associated with the development of ANV, 3) elucidation of the etiological process that underlies the development of ANV, and 4) development and evaluation of behavioral techniques for controlling ANV.

Prevalence of ANV

Nearly two dozen studies have reported prevalence rates for ANV in cancer chemotherapy patients (Burish and Carey 1986) (Table 5–1). In considering the prevalence of ANV, it is important to distinguish between patients who experience anticipatory nausea and those who experience anticipatory vomiting (presumably, but not always, accompanied by nausea). The former is far more common. Prevalence estimates for anticipatory nausea have ranged from 18% (Nicholas 1982) to 57% (Andrykowski et al. 1988), whereas rates for anticipatory vomiting have ranged from 9% (Morrow et al. 1982) to 33% (Wilcox et al. 1982). In large part, this variation is a function of the conceptual and methodological diversity that has characterized ANV research. Specific investigations have varied in 1) how ANV was defined, 2) how and when the presence of ANV was assessed, and 3) the composition of the research sample examined with respect to cytotoxic and antiemetic drug regimens and disease sites represented (Andrykowski 1986). Each factor can markedly influence the prevalence rate obtained.

Fundamental to the scientific enterprise is a precise and commonly shared definition of a particular phenomenon of interest. Unfortunately, ANV research has been hampered by differences in the way this phenomenon has been defined. In some cases, researchers have failed to specify how they defined ANV (e.g., Weddington et al. 1984). More commonly, however, ANV has been defined as nausea or vomiting that occurs *before any* chemotherapy infusion (e.g., Nicholas 1982; van Komen and Redd 1985). This definition, however, fails to take into account the possibility that these symptoms might be attributable to the

Table 5–1. Summary of studies reporting prevalence of anticipatory nausea and vomiting

Study	Sample size	Anticipatory nausea (%)	Anticipatory vomiting (%)	Anticipatory nausea and\or vomiting (%)
Andrykowski et al. 1985	71	37		
Andrykowski et al. 1988	77	57		
Dobkin et al.1985	125	32	12	
Dolgin et al. 1985	80	29	20	
Fetting et al. 1983	123	17	14	
Ingle et al. 1984	60			25
Morrow 1982	225			21
Morrow et al. 1982	406	24	9	
Nerenz et al. 1986	61	24		
Nesse et al. 1980	18	44		
Nicholas 1982	71			18
Olafsdottir et al. 1986	50	40	14	
Scogna and Smalley 1979	41			27
Stefanek et al. 1988	121	15	11	
van Komen and Redd 1985	100	33	11	
Weddington et al. 1984	50			38
Wilcox et al. 1982	52		33	

emetic effect of recent oral or intravenous medication. Because interest in ANV stems largely from its nonpharmacological nature, ANV should be defined so as to exclude instances of pretreatment nausea or vomiting that are attributable to pharmacological or physiological factors. Although this can be accomplished in various ways (e.g., Fetting et al. 1983; Morrow 1982; Nerenz et al. 1982), restriction of the definition of ANV to nausea and/or vomiting experienced before an infusion on Day 1 of a new treatment cycle is recommended (Andrykowski 1986, 1988). This definition usually ensures that the patient has not received any oral or intravenous cytotoxic medications for at least the preceding week. Although not guaranteeing the elimination of physiological or pharmacological confounds, this definition greatly reduces their likelihood.

The methods and timing of assessment of ANV have varied widely across investigations. For example, ANV has been assessed by asking patients via interview or questionnaire whether or not they have ever experienced anticipatory symptoms (e.g., Andrykowski et al. 1985; Morrow 1982; van Komen and Redd 1985). Use of such self-reports is subject to all the biases inherent in asking individuals to report the occurrence and intensity of unpleasant experiences. ANV has been assessed by review of patients' medical records (e.g., Wilcox et al. 1982). This technique is likely to yield lower prevalence estimates, particularly for anticipatory nausea, because medical staff may not be aware of the presence of these symptoms unless patients volunteer this information. Direct observation of ANV has never been used to ascertain the prevalence of these symptoms, although it was used in an intervention study (Redd et al. 1982) to assess the presence of anticipatory vomiting. Although it is useful for assessing vomiting, direct observation is not an appropriate method for assessing the more private and subjective experience of nausea. Until a physiological technique for assessing nausea is developed, self-report will remain the best method for obtaining accurate estimates of ANV prevalence.

The timing of the assessment of ANV has also varied across research studies. Most studies have assessed these symptoms at only one point during the course of chemotherapy treatment. Assessment has occurred after the completion of a fixed number of treatments or cycles for all patients (e.g., Morrow 1982) or at a single point in time for all patients (e.g., Fetting et al. 1983; van Komen and Redd 1985). In the latter case, patients will vary with respect to the number of cycles or treatments received at the time of assessment. The difficulty with one-time assessments is that the likelihood that a patient will experience ANV generally increases with increasing exposure to chemotherapy (Fetting et al. 1983; Nerenz et al. 1986; Olafsdottir et al. 1986). Thus lower prevalence rates will likely be obtained if assessment of ANV occurs relatively early in the course of treatment for most patients, and higher prevalence rates will likely result if assessment occurs later in the course of chemotherapy.

Finally, most studies from which ANV prevalence rates have been obtained have employed heterogenous samples with respect to diagnoses and drug regimens (e.g., Andrykowski et al. 1985; Morrow 1982; van Komen and Redd 1985). Cancer diagnosis is associated with choice of drug regimen and drug regimens vary in their emeticity, which is associated with the likelihood that a patient will develop ANV. For example, Andrykowski et al. (1985) reported that only 20% of patients receiving fluorouracil (a mildly emetic drug) developed ANV, whereas 80% of patients receiving a more emetic regimen consisting of cyclophosphamide, doxorubicin, vincristine, and prednisone did so. In general, higher prevalence rates will characterize research samples that contain a larger proportion of highly toxic regimens. A related factor that will affect ANV prevalence rates, but that is typically neglected in research reports, is the pattern of prescription and use of antiemetic agents characteristic of a study sample. Physicians vary in the types of antiemetic regimens prescribed, with some drugs, routes, and schedules of administration more effective than others in controlling PNV. Moreover, patients vary in the manner in which they use the antiemetics prescribed for them. For example, Andrykowski and Garrison (1989) reported that most patients in a chemotherapy clinic used antiemetics on an as-needed basis rather than on a prophylactic basis. Prophylactic use of antiemetics is generally a more effective means of controlling PNV. ANV prevalence rates will therefore tend to be lower in samples characterized by more effective prescription and usage of antiemetic medications.

In summary, the prevalence of ANV will be influenced by 1) how ANV is defined, 2) at what point and how often during chemotherapy treatment patients are assessed for the presence of ANV, 3) the source(s) of information used to determine the presence of ANV, 4) the emetic profile of each chemotherapy regimen, and 5) the use of antiemetic drugs.

Factors Associated With the Development of ANV

Because not all chemotherapy patients develop ANV, determination of the patient-, disease-, and treatment-related correlates of ANV has been a major research focus. At minimum, this information can be used to identify patients who are at risk for developing ANV as well as to guide intervention efforts aimed at preventing ANV (Burish et al. 1987). In addition, this information can contribute to understanding the biobehavioral processes underlying acquisition of anticipatory symptoms.

Despite the large number of studies that have contrasted patients with and without ANV, the factors related to the development of ANV are still incompletely understood (Table 5–2). By far the most significant factor in differentiating these two groups of patients is the extent

Table 5–2.   Relationships of age, posttreatment nausea and vomiting (PNV), and anxiety to development of anticipatory nausea and vomiting (ANV)

Study	Age	PNV	Anxiety
Altmaier et al. 1982			+
Andrykowski et al. 1985	−	+	+
Andrykowski et al. 1988	−	+	−
Dobkin et al. 1985		+	
Dolgin et al. 1985	+	+	+[a]
Fetting et al. 1983	+	+	
Ingle et al. 1984	+	+	+
Morrow 1982	+	+	
Nerenz et al. 1986	+	+	+
Nesse et al. 1980		+	
Nicholas 1982		+	
Stefanek et al. 1988		+	
van Komen and Redd 1985		+	+
Weddington et al. 1984	+	+	
Wilcox et al. 1982		+	

Note.   + = related to development of ANV; − = not related to development of ANV.
[a]Parent anxiety (pediatric patients).

of PNV experienced: patients with a greater duration, severity, frequency, and/or consistency of PNV are more likely to develop ANV (Andrykowski et al. 1985, 1988; Cohen et al. 1986; Dobkin et al. 1985; Dolgin et al. 1985; Fetting et al. 1983; Morrow 1982, 1984; Nerenz et al. 1986; Nicholas 1982; van Komen and Redd 1985; Weddington et al. 1984). Beyond this assertion, however, little can be stated with confidence. Other variables that have been associated with ANV include increased susceptibility to motion sickness (Morrow 1985); awareness of tastes or odors during infusions (Fetting et al. 1985; Nerenz et al. 1986); age, with younger patients at increased risk for ANV (Cohen et al. 1986; Fetting et al. 1983; Morrow 1982; Nerenz et al. 1986); lengthier infusions (Andrykowski et al. 1985); greater autonomic sensitivity (Olafsdottir et al. 1986); expectations for experiencing chemotherapy-related nausea (Andrykowski et al. 1988); and increased trait anxiety (van Komen and Redd 1985), state anxiety, and general "emotional distress" (Altmaier et al. 1982; Andrykowski et al. 1985; Ingle et al. 1984; Nerenz et al. 1986). Firm conclusions regarding the relationships of these variables to ANV are precluded because each variable has either been examined in only one study or has been found in at least one study not to be related to ANV (Burish and Carey 1986).

Etiology of ANV

Although other explanations have been suggested (Burish and Carey 1986; Redd et al. 1985), the classical (or Pavlovian) conditioning explanation for the development of ANV has achieved wide acceptance. ANV is strikingly similar to the subclass of classical conditioning known as Pavlovian B conditioning (Grant 1964) (Figure 5–1). The

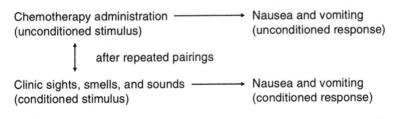

Figure 5–1. Classical conditioning model of anticipatory nausea and vomiting.

reference paradigm for this subclass of classical conditioning involves an animal given repeated injections of morphine. The pharmacological response to morphine involves severe nausea and vomiting and profuse salivation. After repeated daily injections, animals evidence these symptoms at the first touch of the experimenter (Collins and Tatum 1925; Pavlov 1927). In terms of the traditional terminology associated with classical conditioning, infusion of cytotoxic drugs, a complex physiological stimulus (unconditioned stimulus [UCS]), may result in the occurrence of nausea and/or vomiting (unconditioned response [UCR]). Repeated pairing of stimuli (e.g., visual, olfactory, and gustatory) associated with the chemotherapy treatment environment (conditioned stimulus [CS]) may ultimately enable these stimuli alone to elicit symptoms of nausea and/or vomiting (conditioned response [CR]).

It should be noted that recent reformulations of the classical conditioning process as involving the learning of relationships among events (Rescorla 1988) are also able to account for the development of ANV. In this view, patients learn that a consistent relationship exists between going to the clinic and subsequently experiencing nausea and vomiting. Support for the conditioning model of ANV comes from several sources, including research on factors related to the development of ANV, the similarity of ANV to other classically conditioned phenomena, and the inability of any other explanation to suitably account for the observed properties of ANV.

In general, research on the correlates of ANV is consistent with the classical conditioning model in suggesting the importance of PNV in accounting for the presence of ANV in an individual. Simply put, patients who do not experience PNV do not develop ANV. Among those with PNV, the likelihood of developing ANV reliably increases as the frequency, severity, and duration of these symptoms increase (all of which are positively related, although not perfectly, with the emeticity of a particular chemotherapy regimen). This pattern of results is consistent with classical conditioning theory and laboratory research, which suggests that conditioning is facilitated by increased intensity of the UCS and/or UCR (Dragoin 1971; Nachman and Ashe 1973). Furthermore, most other variables that have been found to characterize patients with ANV also support the classical conditioning model. For example, susceptibility to motion sickness likely contributes to ANV development by increasing the likelihood and magnitude of PNV. Lengthier infusions and the experience of infusion-related taste sensations also fit the classical conditioning model (Andrykowski 1987; Andrykowski et al. 1985) because gastrointestinal conditioning is known to be facilitated when the temporal interval between the UCS and UCR is shortened (Garcia et al. 1966) or bridged by distinct gustatory sensations (Best et al. 1985).

Two other explanations have been offered to account for the occurrence of ANV. Neither explanation invokes the classical conditioning process described above. The first explanation attributes ANV to underlying psychological readjustment associated with life-threatening illness with anticipatory symptoms symbolizing rejection of the diagnosis of cancer and the need for chemotherapy treatment (Chang 1981). Arguing against this explanation is the lack of research findings identifying a pattern of psychological maladjustment or psychopathology in patients with ANV. A second explanation notes that gastrointestinal distress can be a concomitant of the stress response (Frain and Valiga 1979; Swanson et al. 1976) and suggests that ANV stems directly from infusion-related anxiety and emotional distress. Because ANV and anxiety frequently coincide (e.g., Altmaier et al. 1982; Ingle et al. 1984; Nerenz et al. 1982; van Komen and Redd 1985), the anxiety hypothesis is appealing. In fact, attribution of ANV to "nerves" is common among patients, family members, and physicians alike (Dolgin et al. 1985; Morrow 1982; Nesse et al. 1980). At a minimum, demonstration that ANV is a simple concomitant of anxiety requires that elevated anxiety levels precede or else coincide with the initial onset of ANV.

The observed relationships between anxiety and ANV onset are complex and contradictory. Nerenz et al. (1986) found that the presence of anxiety before the initial chemotherapy infusion was significantly related to the occurrence of ANV during the first six cycles of treatment. On the other hand, Andrykowski et al. (1988) found that anxiety at the initial infusion was unrelated to the subsequent occurrence of ANV. Andrykowski and Redd (1987) found that anxiety levels for patients who developed ANV early in their course of treatment did not differ from those evidenced by patients who did not develop ANV, leading them to conclude that elevated anxiety was not necessary for the development of ANV. It also should be noted that anxiety levels are generally elevated before a patient's initial infusion, decreasing somewhat with subsequent infusions (Andrykowski et al. 1985). Nevertheless, despite high initial levels of anxiety, not one patient in either of the completely prospective studies of ANV (Andrykowski et al. 1985,

1988) reported nausea or vomiting before their initial infusion.

Other evidence regarding the role of anxiety comes from a pilot study (Fetting et al. 1987) in which patients with ANV received clonidine for 5 days before chemotherapy. Clonidine reduces noradrenergic activity and possesses anxiolytic properties. Four of the eight patients who received clonidine reported that, although PNV persisted, anticipatory symptoms did not recur. The authors carefully noted that the observed effects could have been attributable to factors other than pharmacological activity (e.g., placebo effect and inconsistent occurrence of ANV). Moreover, the relationship between clonidine, noradrenergic activity, and physiological and psychological manifestations of anxiety with ANV remains to be investigated.

Alprazolam has also been studied for its effectiveness against ANV (Greenberg et al. 1987). Patients were administered 0.25 mg of alprazolam at dinner the night before chemotherapy, followed by 0.5 mg at bedtime, 0.5 mg on morning awakening, and 1 mg at noon just before chemotherapy. After chemotherapy, they continued taking 0.5 mg qid for 2 days. This regimen was alternated with a placebo regimen during another cycle of chemotherapy. Results indicated that alprazolam significantly reduced ANV compared with placebo. It should be noted that alprazolam use was not associated with significant reductions in anxiety, arguing against the hypothesis that the observed effects were due solely to anxiety reduction.

In sum, no clear evidence confirms the hypothesis that ANV is simply a physiological concomitant of the stress response. Nor does it appear that patients who develop ANV can be identified early in the course of treatment strictly on the basis of elevated anxiety levels. This does not mean that anxiety does not contribute to the etiology of ANV. Anxiety almost certainly contributes to the development of ANV, at least for some patients. However, although speculation about the potential relationship between anxiety and ANV abounds (Burish and Carey 1986; Redd et al. 1985), empirical support for most hypotheses is lacking. At this juncture, it appears most reasonable to conclude that anxiety facilitates the development of ANV by exacerbating the degree of PNV experienced (Jacobsen et al. 1988), with the latter being the primary factor leading to the classical conditioning of ANV. In particular, this process might describe the etiology of ANV among patients who develop these symptoms relatively late in their course of treatment (Andrykowski and Redd 1987; Andrykowski et al. 1988).

Management of ANV

Clinical Outcomes

Although research evidence is absent regarding the utility of antiemetic medications in controlling ANV, clinical reports suggest that these symptoms are generally refractory to pharmacological intervention (Chang 1981; Redd et al. 1982). As a result, a variety of behavioral techniques have been used to control ANV (Table 5–3). The techniques that have been most extensively evaluated include 1) hypnosis, 2) progressive muscle relaxation (PMR) with guided imagery, 3) systematic desensitization, and 4) distraction. Other techniques that have shown promise, but have appeared in only a single case report, include stimulus control (i.e., taste blocking [Greene and Seime 1987]) and multiple-site electromyographic biofeedback and relaxation (Burish et al. 1981).

Although antiemetics are unlikely to eliminate ANV once it has developed, the prophylactic use of antiemetics could serve to prevent anticipatory symptoms from ever developing. Conditioning theory pos-

Table 5–3. Behavioral management of anticipatory nausea and vomiting

Study	Intervention	Outcome
Burish et al. 1987	Progressive muscle relaxation and guided (prophylactic intervention)	Anticipatory nausea reduced; anxiety reduced
Lyles et al. 1982	Progressive muscle relaxation and guided imagery	Anticipatory nausea reduced; anxiety reduced
Morrow and Morrell 1982	Systematic desensitization	Anticipatory nausea and vomiting reduced; no change in anxiety
Redd et al. 1982	Hypnosis	Anticipatory vomiting eliminated
Redd et al. 1987	Cognitive distraction	Anticipatory nausea reduced; no change in anxiety

tulates that a conditioned response can only occur if an unconditioned response is present. Thus if antiemetic treatment successfully prevents PNV, ANV should not develop. Research evidence supports this point. Two separate studies have reported that among patients who developed ANV, every individual had at least one prior episode of PNV (Andrykowski et al. 1985, 1988). There are also reasons to believe that ANV can be prevented or its intensity limited if antiemetic drugs limit PNV to very low levels. As previously discussed, research evidence indicates that patients who experience less severe PNV are less likely to develop ANV. Moreover, conditioning theory suggests that the intensity of a conditioned side effect, at least when it initially develops, does not exceed the intensity of the corresponding unconditioned side effect. Thus even if ANV develops, it should be of mild intensity if PNV has been limited to very low levels.

The first behavioral technique to be investigated as a means of controlling chemotherapy-related nausea and vomiting was hypnosis. Early reports focused largely on the use of this procedure with children and suggested its utility in controlling gastrointestinal symptoms (Dash 1980; Dempster et al. 1976; LaBaw et al. 1975; Olness 1981). Unfortunately, this research suffered from failure to 1) adequately describe the intervention procedures used, 2) distinguish the control of PNV from the control of ANV, and 3) rigorously measure clinical outcomes.

The only controlled outcome study of the effectiveness of hypnosis in controlling ANV is that of Redd et al. (1982). Six patients who had displayed anticipatory vomiting before at least three consecutive infusions served as subjects. An individual-analysis, multiple-baseline research design was used. After two training sessions held outside the clinic, therapist-directed hypnosis, in conjunction with guided imagery, was used before and during chemotherapy infusions. (For a more detailed description of the intervention procedures, see Redd et al. 1982.) The results revealed that whenever the intervention was employed, all patients evidenced decreases in nausea before and during chemotherapy and complete elimination of anticipatory vomiting. The power of hypnosis and imagery in controlling ANV was further illustrated when, because of scheduling difficulties, three patients chose to undergo chemotherapy treatment without the intervention. On these occasions, their ANV returned. The ANV was again eliminated when hypnosis and imagery were reinstituted during subsequent infusions.

A series of studies using PMR and guided imagery to control ANV has been completed by Burish and colleagues (Burish and Lyles 1979, 1981; Lyles et al. 1982). The methods they used have been similar in each study. Adults with ANV were studied across 5 to 10 consecutive infusions divided into baseline, intervention, and follow-up phases. Pre- and postinfusion measures of pulse rate, blood pressure, anxiety, and depression were obtained. Patient and nurse ratings of nausea during infusions, as well as nurses' observations of vomiting, were obtained after each infusion. After the baseline phase, a therapist directed patients in PMR and guided relaxation imagery both before and during infusions. The relaxation procedure he or she employed is similar to Redd et al.'s hypnotic procedure (1982). Although differing in how relaxation is initially induced, both used therapist-guided imagery of tranquil scenes to increase relaxation. During the follow-up phase, patients used PMR and imagery on their own both before and during infusions. In two studies (Burish and Lyles 1981; Lyles et al. 1982), no-treatment and therapist-contact control groups were added to assess the contribution of nonspecific factors to treatment outcomes. Results have been consistent across their research. During the intervention phase, PMR and guided imagery produced reductions in pulse rate, blood pressure, and self-reports of anxiety and nausea. Patients in control conditions did not evidence these reductions. Results during the follow-up phase were less impressive. Reductions in nausea and physiological arousal were not as marked when the therapist was no longer present to direct the patient through the PMR and imagery intervention.

Systematic desensitization has also been used to control ANV (Morrow and Morrell 1982). In this research, adult patients were assigned to one of three groups: systematic desensitization, standard counseling (involving a problem-solving and support approach), or a no-treatment control group. Patients in the systematic desensitization and counseling groups participated in two 1-hour treatment sessions between their fourth and fifth infusions. In the desensitization group, hierarchies were individualized to some extent for each patient but typically began with scenes describing the patient entering the waiting room for treatment. Patient ratings of the frequency, severity, and duration of ANV were obtained for two follow-up infusions. Results revealed that systematic desensitization was superior to both counseling and no-treatment in reducing the frequency, severity, and duration of anticipatory nausea and the severity of anticipatory vomiting.

Cognitive-attentional distraction, operationalized as the playing of commercially available video games, has also been employed as a means of controlling ANV. Redd et al. (1987) studied 15 pediatric patients with ANV using a design that incorporated multiple baseline and intervention phases. Following a no-video-game baseline assessment, patients played a video game for 10 minutes, followed by a 10-minute no-video-game period and then by a second 10-minute video game period. Self-reports of nausea and anxiety as well as measures of pulse rate and blood pressure were obtained from each patient at the conclusion of each of the four study phases. Results indicated that nausea was significantly reduced during the two video game phases, relative to the two baseline phases. The pattern of results for anxiety was similar but did not attain statistical significance. Finally, physiological indices were not altered consistently by the presentation or withdrawal of the video game intervention.

In addition to its clinical utility, the video game intervention sheds light on the theoretical debate concerning mechanisms underlying the effectiveness of behavioral interventions in controlling ANV (Lyles et al. 1982; Redd and Andrykowski 1982). Whereas hypnosis, PMR and guided imagery, and, to a lesser degree, systematic desensitization all combine elements of distraction with relaxation, video games presumably use distraction alone. Thus the results reported by Redd et al. (1987) are theoretically significant insofar as they suggest that reductions in ANV can be attained with a suitable distracting task, independent of physiological relaxation and anxiety reduction.

Clinical Issues

In general, the above discussion strongly suggests that behavioral intervention can be effective in reducing or eliminating ANV in both adult and pediatric patients. However, several issues arise regarding the clinical implementation of these interventions, including 1) selecting among available techniques, 2) maximizing cost-effectiveness, and 3) managing resistance to behavioral intervention.

Selecting which intervention to use with a particular patient is difficult because no direct comparison of the relative efficacy of behavioral interventions in controlling ANV has been conducted. Because of their similarity, it is particularly difficult to choose between hypnosis (Redd et al. 1982) and PMR with guided imagery (Burish and Lyles

1981). Procedurally, these two techniques differ primarily with respect to the manner in which relaxation is initially induced. Redd induced relaxation passively with direct suggestions of warmth, comfort, and heaviness, whereas Burish induced relaxation actively through sequential tensing and relaxing of various muscle groups. As a result, PMR plus imagery might be contraindicated for the weak or debilitated patient for whom muscle tension may be painful. Nominally, the Redd technique is labeled "hypnosis" whereas the Burish technique is not, a consideration that should not be minimized. Misunderstanding and fear of hypnosis is relatively commonplace and may result in some patients refusing to participate in an intervention referred to as "hypnosis" (Hendler and Redd 1985). On the other hand, some patients may derive greater benefits if an intervention is described as "hypnosis" because it may encourage more positive expectations regarding potential benefits (Redd and Andrykowski 1982). Straightforward discussion of the patient's beliefs and expectations regarding available techniques should be encouraged and this information should be used to guide selection of an intervention strategy. The following case example illustrates many of these points:

Case 1

Mr. P, a 35-year-old man being treated for Hodgkin's disease, was referred for psychiatric consultation by his oncologist because of complaints that he felt extremely anxious and nauseated during chemotherapy treatment. These symptoms had not responded to an increase in dosage of his antiemetic medication (Compazine). At the initial interview conducted between chemotherapy treatments, he provided the following history. He had received two infusions of cytotoxic chemotherapy and had tolerated them well. However, following the third infusion, he experienced significant PNV. Before the next infusion, he reported that he became "sweaty and queasy" on arriving in the waiting area. Before the most recent infusion, he reported that he became nauseated on entering the hospital. He also stated that, as the needle was inserted to start chemotherapy, he vomited. He expressed considerable embarrassment and distress over these symptoms. Although he felt he could tolerate the posttreatment side effects, he was not sure whether he would be able to complete the scheduled number of infusions if the anticipatory symptoms persisted.

Mr. P's history revealed no indications of past or present psychiatric disorder. Based on his description of his symptoms, his condition was diagnosed as ANV. Treatment was initiated during the initial interview by first providing him with an explanation of how his condition had arisen. This explanation emphasized that 1) his anticipatory symptoms were a normal reaction to chemotherapy and experienced by many patients, 2) the symptoms arose through a conditioning process by which associations were formed between coming to the clinic and subsequently experiencing gastrointestinal distress, and 3) often these symptoms can be reduced or eliminated by learning relaxation skills and using them in the period before chemotherapy administration. The therapist then conducted a brief relaxation exercise with him in the office. During this exercise, the therapist instructed Mr. P in how to shift attention away from environmental cues by focusing on his breathing and in how to achieve a measure of relaxation by attending to the therapist's suggestions. In addition, the therapist worked with him to construct a relaxing visual image.

Mr. P was able to imagine a beach scene in which he "could almost feel" the warmth of the sun and could breathe in unison with the gentle motion of the waves. The therapist tape-recorded the relaxation exercise for him and asked him to practice the exercise once each day during the 5 days before the next infusion. The therapist also instructed him to listen to the tape on the way into the hospital (using a portable cassette player and headphones). Finally, the therapist arranged to see him in an office away from the chemotherapy treatment area just before the next infusion.

On the day of the infusion, Mr. P arrived at the therapist's office in a relaxed state, listening to the audiotape. A much abbreviated version of the previous exercise was conducted, and then Mr. P and the therapist proceeded to the chemotherapy clinic. The chemotherapy was administered without incident with Mr. P experiencing a strong sense of relief and accomplishment. He completed his chemotherapy as scheduled and with continued success, using the audiotape before each treatment. He reported that as he became adept in the relaxation exercise he would "tune out" the tape and focus on his self-generated image of the beach. He also reported that the relaxation exercise was useful as a means of inducing sleep at bedtime. Mr. P and his oncologist expressed their satisfaction with the behavioral treatment.

At present, the cost of providing behavioral treatment for ANV is high. With the exception of video games, all of the interventions described above use a therapist with specialized training to administer the intervention. The amount of therapist time involvement is often

substantial, yet the research clearly indicates that effectiveness is max-
imized by having a trained therapist implement the techniques (Carey
and Burish 1987; Lyles et al. 1982; Redd et al. 1982). Specific suggestions for reducing the labor intensiveness of implementing hypnosis or
PMR with guided imagery have been advanced (Jacobsen and Redd
1988; Redd and Andrykowski 1982). These include training nonprofes-
sionals (e.g., nursing staff, spouses, and relatives) to implement these
techniques or explicitly encouraging patient self-administration of
these techniques through gradual "fading" of therapist involvement or
the use of an audiotaped intervention. Although clinical experience
suggests that these innovations can work well for some patients, for
many patients it is difficult to achieve or maintain clinically significant
reductions in ANV in the absence of concerted therapist involvement.
Research investigating how these techniques can best be adapted to
increase availability would be of value. However, the present lack of
such research is probably a good barometer of the real difficulties
involved in attempting to minimize therapist involvement while simultaneously maximizing clinical benefit.

Resistance to the use of behavioral interventions for controlling
ANV can assume a variety of forms. As discussed above, some patients
may refuse "hypnotic" interventions. More common, perhaps, are patients who are interested in behavioral intervention but are reluctant to
invest the amount of time necessary to master the techniques. For
example, home practice is an integral aspect of both hypnosis (Redd et
al. 1982) and PMR with guided imagery (Burish and Lyles 1981), yet
patients will occasionally fail to practice, thus limiting treatment benefits (in addition to frustrating their therapist). As explanation, patients
often indicate that home practice (e.g., listening to an audiotape of their
intervention) is aversive because it reminds them that they have cancer
and require aversive chemotherapy treatments. However, as Jacobsen
and Redd (1988) have indicated, such patients can still derive benefit
from listening to an audiotaped intervention while they are at the clinic
or in the hospital.

In other instances, the failure to practice stems from a lack of
agreement between the patient and therapist regarding the roles of each.
The intent of home practice is to allow patients to develop the skills
necessary to conduct the intervention on their own during chemotherapy. Some patients, however, may not embrace this goal, preferring
that the therapist always be present to deliver the intervention. Clini-

cians should be sensitive to this issue, and explicitly discuss with the patient their mutual roles as well as the goals of behavioral intervention. These issues should be clarified at the beginning of therapy and further discussed as necessary throughout the patient's course of chemotherapy.

Finally, resistance to behavioral intervention may occasionally stem from medical staff. In most instances this resistance results from lack of familiarity with behaviorally oriented clinicians and techniques. Often this resistance stems from concern that the clinician might usurp the close relationship that the oncologist or primary nurse has with the patient. To combat these concerns, it is important to emphasize to medical staff that behavioral intervention is an adjunct to the patient's routine therapy and that the behavioral clinician is prepared to function as a member of the health care team. Once initial concerns are allayed, medical staff are typically receptive to behavioral intervention. In part this is due to recognition that the behavioral approach is compatible with medical oncology with regard to problem diagnosis and treatment evaluation. Like medical oncology, behavioral intervention focuses on concrete, objectively measurable problems; individualizes treatment in accordance with changes in patient behavior; and is empirical, rather than theoretical, in its orientation.

Summary

In this chapter, we have reviewed the literature on the etiology and treatment of ANV. The key points that can be gleaned from this literature are that 1) ANV is a relatively common symptom in cancer chemotherapy patients, 2) ANV arises through a process of conditioned learning, and 3) patients who develop ANV are more likely to have received more emetic chemotherapy and/or to have experienced worse PNV. Finally, three techniques hold promise for reducing or eliminating ANV: 1) effective antiemetic control of PNV, 2) the use of anxiolytic drugs such as clonidine and alprazolam, and 3) the use of behavioral techniques that involve distraction and relaxation.

References

Altmaier EM, Ross WE, Moore K: A pilot investigation of the psychologic function of patients with anticipatory vomiting. Cancer 49:201–204, 1982

Andrykowski MA: Definitional issues in the study of anticipatory nausea in cancer chemotherapy. J Behav Med 9: 33–41, 1986

Andrykowski MA: Do infusion-related tastes and odors facilitate the development of anticipatory nausea? a failure to support hypothesis. Health Psychol 6:329–341, 1987

Andrykowski MA: Defining anticipatory nausea and vomiting: Differences among cancer chemotherapy patients who report pretreatment nausea. J Behav Med 11:59–69, 1988

Andrykowski MA, Garrison J: Prescription and use of antiemetics among cancer chemotherapy outpatients. Journal of Psychosocial Oncology 7:141–158, 1989

Andrykowski MA, Redd WH: Longitudinal analysis of the development of anticipatory nausea. J Consult Clin Psychol 55:36–41, 1987

Andrykowski MA, Redd WH, Hatfield AK: Development of anticipatory nausea: a prospective analysis. J Consult Clin Psychol 53:447–454, 1985

Andrykowski MA, Jacobsen PB, Marks E, et al: Prevalence, predictors, and course of anticipatory nausea in women receiving adjuvant chemotherapy for breast cancer. Cancer 62:2607–2613, 1988

Best MR, Batson JD, Meachum CL, et al: Characteristics of taste-mediated environmental potentiation in rats. Learning and Motivation 16:190–209, 1985

Burish TG, Carey MP: Conditioned aversive responses in cancer chemotherapy patients: theoretical and developmental analysis. J Consult Clin Psychol 54:593–600, 1986

Burish TG, Lyles JN: Effectiveness of relaxation training in reducing the aversiveness of chemotherapy in the treatment of cancer. J Behav Ther Exp Psychiatry 10:357–361, 1979

Burish TG, Lyles JN: Effectiveness of relaxation training in reducing adverse reactions to cancer chemotherapy. J Behav Med 4:65–78, 1981

Burish TG, Shartner CD, Lyles JN: Effectiveness of multiple muscle-site EMG biofeedback and relaxation training in reducing the aversiveness of cancer chemotherapy. Biofeedback Self Regul 6:523–535, 1981

Burish TG, Carey MP, Krozely MG, et al: Conditioned side effects induced by cancer chemotherapy: prevention through behavioral treatment. J Consult Clin Psychol 55:42–48, 1987

Carey MP, Burish TG: Providing relaxation training to cancer chemotherapy patients: a comparison of three delivery techniques. J Consult Clin Psychol 55:732–737, 1987

Carey MP, Burish TG: Etiology and treatment of the psychological side effects associated with cancer chemotherapy: a critical review and discussion. Psychol Bull 104:307–325, 1988

Chang JC: Nausea and vomiting in cancer patients: an expression of psychological mechanisms. Psychosomatics 22:707–709, 1981

Cohen RE, Blanchard EB, Ruckdeschel JC, et al: Prevalence and correlates of posttreatment and anticipatory nausea and vomiting in cancer chemotherapy. J Psychosom Res 30:643–654, 1986

Collins KH, Tatum AL: A conditioned salivary reflex established by chronic morphine poisoning. Am J Physiol 74:14–15, 1925

Dash J: Hypnosis for symptom amelioration, in Psychological Aspects of Childhood Cancer. Edited by Kellerman J. Springfield, IL, Charles C Thomas, 1980, pp 215–230

Dempster CR, Balson P, Whalen BT: Supportive hypnotherapy during the radical treatment of malignancies. Int J Clin Exp Hypn 24:1–9, 1976

Dobkin P, Zeichner A, Dickson-Parnell B: Concomitants of anticipatory nausea and emesis in cancer patients in chemotherapy. Psychol Rep 56:671–676, 1985

Dolgin MJ, Katz ER, McGinty K, et al: Anticipatory nausea and vomiting in pediatric cancer patients. Pediatrics 75:547–552, 1985

Dragoin WB: Conditioning and extinction of taste aversions with variations in the intensity of the CS and UCS in two strains of rats. Psychonomic Science 22:303–305, 1971

Fetting JH, Wilcox PM, Iwata BA, et al: Anticipatory nausea and vomiting in an ambulatory medical oncology population. Cancer Treat Rep 67:1093–1098, 1983

Fetting JH, Wilcox PM, Sheidler VR, et al: Tastes associated with parenteral chemotherapy for breast cancer. Cancer Treat Rep 69:1249–1251, 1985

Fetting JH, Sheidler VR, Stefanek ME, et al: Clonidine for anticipatory nausea and vomiting: a pilot study examining dose-toxicity relationships and potential for further study. Cancer Treatment Reports 71:409–410, 1987

Frain M, Valiga T: The multiple dimensions of stress. Topics in Clinical Nursing 1:43–52, 1979

Garcia J, Ervin FR, Koelling RA: Learning with prolonged delay of reinforcement. Psychonomic Science 5:121–122, 1966

Grant DA: Classical and operant conditioning, in Categories of Human Learning. Edited by Melton AW. New York, Academic Press, 1964, pp 1–31

Greenberg DB, Surman OS, Clarke J, et al: Alprazolam for phobic nausea and vomiting related to chemotherapy. Cancer Treatment Reports 71:549–550, 1987

Greene PG, Seime RJ: Stimulus control of anticipatory nausea in cancer chemotherapy. J Behav Ther Exp Psychiatry 18:61–64, 1987

Hendler CS, Redd WH: Fear of hypnosis: the role of labeling in patients' acceptance of behavioral interventions. Behavior Therapy 17:2–13, 1985

Ingle RJ, Burish TG, Wallston KA: Conditionability of cancer chemotherapy patients. Oncology Nursing Forum 11:97–102, 1984

Jacobsen PB, Redd WH: The development and management of chemotherapy-related anticipatory nausea and vomiting. Cancer Invest 6:329–336, 1988

Jacobsen PB, Andrykowski MA, Redd WH, et al: Nonpharmacologic factors in the development of posttreatment nausea with adjuvant chemotherapy for breast cancer. Cancer 61:379–385, 1988

LaBaw W, Holton C, Tewell K, et al: The use of self-hypnosis by children with cancer. Am J Clin Hypn 17:233–238, 1975

Lyles JN, Burish TG, Krozely MG, et al: Efficacy of relaxation training and guided imagery in reducing the aversiveness of cancer chemotherapy. J Consult Clin Psychol 50:509–524, 1982

Morrow GR: Prevalence and correlates of anticipatory nausea and vomiting in chemotherapy patients. J Natl Cancer Inst 68:585–588, 1982

Morrow GR: Clinical characteristics associated with the development of anticipatory nausea and vomiting in cancer patients undergoing chemotherapy treatment. J Clin Oncol 2:1170–1176, 1984

Morrow GR: The effect of a susceptibility to motion sickness on the side effects of cancer chemotherapy. Cancer 55:2766–2770, 1985

Morrow GR, Dobkin PL: Anticipatory nausea and vomiting in cancer patients undergoing chemotherapy treatment: prevalence, etiology, and behavioral interventions. Clinical Psychology Review 8:517–556, 1988

Morrow GR, Morrell BS: Behavioral treatment for the anticipatory nausea and vomiting induced by cancer chemotherapy. N Engl J Med 307:1476–1480, 1982

Morrow GR, Arseneau JC, Asbury RF, et al: Anticipatory nausea and vomiting with chemotherapy. N Engl J Med 306:431–432, 1982

Nachman M, Ashe JH: Learned taste aversions in rats as a function of dosage, concentration, and route of administration of LiCl. Physiol Behav 10:73–78, 1973

Nerenz DR, Leventhal H, Love RR: Factors contributing to emotional distress during cancer chemotherapy. Cancer 50:1020–1027, 1982

Nerenz DR, Leventhal H, Easterling DV, et al: Anxiety and drug taste as predictors of anticipatory nausea in cancer chemotherapy. J Clin Oncol 4:224–233, 1986

Nesse RM, Carli T, Curtis GC, et al: Pretreatment nausea in cancer chemotherapy: a conditioned response? Psychosom Med 42:33–36, 1980

Nicholas DR: Prevalence of anticipatory nausea and emesis in cancer chemotherapy patients. J Behav Med 5:461–463, 1982

Olafsdottir M, Sjoden PO, Westling B: Prevalence and prediction of chemotherapy-related anxiety, nausea, and vomiting in cancer patients. Behav Res Ther 24:59–66, 1986

Olness K: Imagery (self-hypnosis) as adjunct therapy in childhood cancer: clinical experience with 25 patients. Am J Pediatr Hematol Oncol 3:313–

321, 1981

Pavlov IP: Conditioned Reflexes: An Investigation of Physiological Activity of the Cerebral Cortex (Lecture III). Oxford, England, Oxford University Press, 1927

Redd WH, Andrykowski MA: Behavioral intervention in cancer treatment: controlling aversion reactions to chemotherapy. J Consult Clin Psychol 43:595–600, 1982

Redd WH, Andresen GV, Minagawa RY: Hypnotic control of anticipatory emesis in patients receiving cancer chemotherapy. J Consult Clinical Psychol 50:14–19, 1982

Redd WH, Burish TG, Andrykowski MA: Aversive conditioning and cancer chemotherapy, in Cancer, Nutrition, and Eating Behavior: A Biobehavioral Perspective. Edited by Burish TG, Levy SM, Meyerowitz BE. Hillsdale, NJ, Lawrence Earlbaum, 1985, pp 117–132

Redd WH, Jacobsen PB, Die-Trill M, et al: Cognitive/attentional distraction in the control of conditioned nausea in pediatric cancer patients receiving chemotherapy. J Consult Clin Psychol 55:391–395, 1987

Rescorla RA: Pavlovian conditioning: it's not what you think it is. Am Psychol 43:151–160, 1988

Scogna DM, Smalley RV: Chemotherapy-induced nausea and vomiting. Am J Nursing 79:1562–1563, 1979

Stefanek ME, Sheidler VR, Fetting JH: Anticipatory nausea and vomiting: does it remain a significant clinical problem? Cancer 62:2654–2657, 1988

Swanson DW, Swenson WM, Huizenga KA, et al: Persistent nausea without organic cause. Mayo Clin Proc 51:257–262, 1976

van Komen RW, Redd WH: Personality factors associated with anticipatory nausea/vomiting in patients receiving cancer chemotherapy. Health Psychol 4:189–202, 1985

Weddington WW: Psychogenic nausea and vomiting associated with cancer chemotherapy. Psychother Psychosom 37:129–136, 1982

Weddington WW, Miller NJ, Sweet DL: Anticipatory nausea and vomiting associated with cancer chemotherapy. J Psychosom Res 28:73–77, 1984

Wilcox PM, Fetting JH, Nettlesheim KM, et al: Anticipatory vomiting in women receiving cyclophosphamide, methotrexate, and 5-FU (CMF) adjuvant chemotherapy for breast carcinoma. Cancer Treat Rep 66:1601–1604, 1982

Chapter 6

Behavioral Control of Anxiety, Distress, and Learned Aversions in Pediatric Oncology

Kenneth Gorfinkle, Ph.D.
William H. Redd, Ph.D.

*T*reatment for cancer in children is extremely aggressive and can be more painful than the disease itself. Especially stressful are repeated infusions of highly emetic chemotherapeutic agents, bone marrow aspirations, lumbar punctures, and blood tests. In many cases these procedures are continued long after the child has ceased feeling "sick" or has any observable symptoms. Because of the anxiety and pain caused by such invasive treatment and many children's lack of understanding, young patients often become noncompliant and actively resist (Jay 1988). Moreover, the distress these children feel is typically made worse by the anxiety their parents display (Jay et al. 1983; Johnson and Baldwin 1968; Wright and Alpern 1981).

Although pharmacological interventions to reduce pain and anxiety in pediatric oncology patients are available, there have been few empirical tests of their effectiveness. Furthermore, the physical risks of commonly used anesthetics and analgesics often outweigh the possible benefits. Risks include central nervous system toxicity, respiratory depression, and liver and kidney toxicity. In addition to the possible physical complications, many children find the experience of receiving these agents aversive. Interviews with pediatric patients (Andrykowski and Redd 1987) have revealed a frequent unwillingness to be regularly sedated. Another pharmacological option is the use of local anesthetics. Two studies (Clarke and Radford 1986; Wahlstedt et al. 1986) have been reported in which a topical cream (eutectic mixture of local anesthetics [EMLA]) was tested in double-blind placebo trials. Research found a reduction of venipuncture pain when cream was used. However, this technique has not received wide usage primarily because it is cumbersome to apply and impractical in clinics in which large numbers of children are treated daily.

Because of these limitations, interest has focused on the use of behavioral techniques to control pain and distress. The major effort has been toward developing multicomponent interventions involving various combinations of the following techniques: 1) positive motivation (reinforcement), 2) attentional distraction, and 3) emotive imagery and hypnosis. In this chapter, we focus on these applications of behavior theory.

Several texts (Burish and Bradley 1983; McGrath and Unruh 1987; Ross and Ross 1988) review research on control of pain in children and adolescents, but the literature on psychological interventions for children undergoing aggressive medical treatment remains limited.

Pain and Distress of Treatment

Cancer treatment often causes more distress than the disease itself and can, at times, resemble torture. Indeed, it is not uncommon for nursing staff to have to restrain pediatric patients during routine venipuncture. One study (Jacobsen et al. 1990) revealed that one-third of children between ages 3 and 7 had to be held down by force to complete the intravenous insertion. Significant anticipatory arousal has also been found; children's emotional distress immediately before routine bone marrow aspiration has been shown to be accompanied by elevated blood pressure and heart rate (Spinetta and Maloney 1975). Koocher and Sallan (1978) aptly observed that "patients are often uncertain as to whether the aggressor is the disease or the physician" (p. 283).

Although older children generally show less distress than do younger children and appear to have less anticipatory anxiety, patients do not habituate by becoming less distressed with repeated injections (Jay et al. 1983). In the case of patients receiving chemotherapy, repeated infusions can lead to phobic-like conditioned aversion responses (Andrykowski and Redd 1987; Redd and Andrykowski 1982; van Komen and Redd 1985). (For a thorough discussion of this phenomenon, see Chapter 5.) The prevalence of such responses in a sample of 80 children receiving emetigenic chemotherapy for a wide variety of cancer diagnoses was at least 28% (Dolgin et al. 1985). Unfortunately, these symptoms do not extinguish or disappear readily; they can last for years. In follow-up interviews with individuals who were cured of leukemia or Hodgkin's disease as children, the former patients often reported that they still felt nauseated whenever they entered the hospital or smelled rubbing alcohol (Cella and Tross 1986). The same study reported one Hodgkin's disease survivor's statement that he could still vividly recall the chemotherapy infusions he received 12 years earlier and that the thought of them still made him nauseated. Although this case does not represent a uniform pattern, it does demonstrate the powerful impact that treatment can have on patients' behavior and attitudes.

A spectrum of treatment-related distress reactions can be identified. Children may experience 1) anxiety in anticipation of invasive treatment, 2) pain and anxiety during immediate treatment (e.g., the pain of the needle and the sensation of the aspiration), 3) conditioned anticipatory reactions (e.g., nausea and vomiting) with chemotherapy, and 4) phobic reactions to the treatment environment (e.g., needles and intravenous bottles). Almost all pediatric patients experience the immediate distress of treatment and many experience all four.

Factors Influencing Children's Reactions to Invasive Medical Procedures

Children's emotional reactions to medical procedures vary widely; some children begin crying loudly as the nurse cleans the skin for routine blood tests, whereas others sit stoically. The factors that determine the nature and intensity of children's reactions have only recently been systematically studied. Age of the child is clearly relevant. Research has shown that the level of distress is 5 to 10 times greater in children less than 7 years old (Jay et al. 1983). Not only are younger children generally poorer at impulse control (depending on the age of the pediatric patient, equivalent levels of aversive stimulation evoke different magnitudes of expressed distress), they may also fail to understand why the procedures are being done. Younger children often think that doctors and nurses are punishing them for some wrong deed (Katz et al. 1980). Moreover, many children believe that they can die from the procedures (Jay 1988; Spinetta and Maloney 1975). These misattributions regarding the cause of illness and the effect of treatment appear to be related to younger children's level of cognitive development (Perrin and Gerrity 1981).

Role of Parents

It has been shown that parents play an important role in modulating children's expressions of emotional distress. Parental anxiety, for example, has been found to be positively correlated with children's distress during painful medical procedures (Jay et al. 1983; Johnson and Baldwin 1968; Wright and Alpern 1981), with children's self-reported hospital fears, and with the severity of the medical condition (Dolgin et al. 1989).

In the face of threat and uncertainty, young children look to their parents for emotional support and for guidance in understanding what is happening. Children are keenly aware of their parents' reactions and quickly respond to any signs of anxiety on the parents' part. Parental tone of voice, posture, and eye gaze are subtle but powerful cues for children during stressful events (Bloom 1975). If the parents are calm and relaxed, the children may be more likely to believe that the situation is safe. If, on the other hand, the parents are clearly anxious and out of control, the children's anxiety is fueled. Research suggests that a complex feedback loop exists between parent and child, with each being exquisitely sensitive to the other's emotional reaction (Bloom 1977). This observation is supported by research in medical sociology (Mechanic 1979), psychoanalytic theory (Freud 1970), and cognitive development (Piaget 1963, 1969).

Research with children undergoing venipuncture indicates that parent-child rapport is critical (Gorfinkle 1988). Parents whose level of coping activity (i.e., distracting, soothing, and explaining) more closely matched their children's level of observed distress during venipuncture subsequently had less distressed children. We have used the term *congruence* to identify this relationship between parent and child behavior (Gorfinkle 1988). We hypothesize that a parent whose behavior does not reflect congruence with the child's distress is perhaps less able to effectively comfort, distract, or soothe the child as the painful part of a procedure approaches. This phenomenon seems to hold true throughout the medical procedure. At an early stage, the parent either succeeds or fails to convey to the child that he or she is responsive to the child's actual level of distress. If the child is quiet and the parent is actively engaging in comforting behavior, the child subsequently becomes more aroused. Thus the parent's careful tracking of the child's general level of arousal appears to be key to effective reduction of child anxiety. Support is lent to the congruence hypothesis by a report (Dolgin et al. 1989) of a significant relationship between children's self-reported fears of the hospital and parents' likelihood of resorting to physical force to control their child.

Controlling Distress and Increasing Patient Compliance

Behavioral interventions (Jay 1988; Manne et al. 1990) developed to alleviate distress during painful medical procedures and encourage compliance with treatment and rehabilitation have generally involved a combination of positive motivation, attentional distraction, emotive imagery, and hypnosis. Distinctions between behavioral, cognitive-behavioral, and hypnotic approaches can become blurred in clinical practice, as interventions are designed to fit particular situations and expertise of the practitioner. Furthermore, as Hendler and Redd (1986) have argued, the strategies share many features such as individualized intervention, explanation of the purpose of proposed interventions, and patient feedback.

Positive Motivation

The goal is to motivate the child to cooperate with parents and medical personnel when unpleasant or painful medical procedures must be performed. The strategy is to present pleasurable consequences when the child behaves appropriately. The most obvious application with pediatric populations is praising desired behavior and providing tangible rewards. In clinical applications with pediatric dental and medical patients, stars and points redeemable for prizes and toy trinkets have been effectively used to increase cooperation during treatment and to encourage compliance with follow-up care.

A critical, and often overlooked, factor in any positive motivation system concerns the value the child places on the rewards that are given. Tokens and points will be ineffective motivators if the child does not value them intrinsically or want the things they buy. Here arises a concept central to behavioral psychology: individualized intervention. If the motivation system is to be effective, it must be tailored to the child. The object or event used as a reward must be seen by the child as fun, interesting, or enjoyable; the child has to want it if it is to function as a motivator.

Positive incentive programs can also be used to motivate the patient to practice the technique that will help control pain and distress. Making rewards contingent on a circumscribed set of behaviors accomplishes two things: 1) the child is ensured a successful experience and 2) the scope of what is required of the child is narrowed to an understandable, realistic level. In the case of cooperating with the nurse during venipuncture, for example, the child is rewarded for holding still and engaging in a simple distraction task, rather than for an amorphous "being good." A specific example is a 6-year-old boy who kicked and cried during routine mouth care; he was so disruptive that three nurses were required to complete the daily procedure. A simple contingency system was initiated: if he did not kick or hit the nurses during mouth care and was generally cooperative, his mother would read him a favorite story. If he actively resisted, two more nurses would be called and he would miss the storybook time with his mother. After 3 days of behavioral intervention his resistance to mouth care was no longer a problem: he was cooperative and proud of his accomplishment. Similar positive incentive programs have been used with pediatric patients to increase compliance with radiation treatment (i.e., special privileges given for holding still) and routine blood tests.

Attentional Distraction

Clinical research with adults has repeatedly demonstrated that anxiety reduction and lowered physiological arousal results in decreased pain intensity (Hilgard and LeBaron 1982, 1984; Kellerman et al. 1983). Moreover, research with adult cancer patients has shown that patients can be trained in specific relaxation techniques to control their own anxiety and thereby reduce pain and distress during invasive medical procedures (Kuttner et al. 1988; Redd et al. 1982; Reeves et al. 1983). Although it appears clear that anxiety plays an equally important role with children, relaxation techniques used with adults are, for the most part, less easily applied with children. For young children who simply cannot sit still, it is unrealistic to ask them to focus their attention on states of muscle relaxation or to go through the muscle exercises required for effective symptom control (Hilgard and LeBaron 1984). A more effective strategy has been to distract the child's attention. Through story telling, fantasy play, and active involvement in an intellectual task (e.g., games) during painful procedures, the child's attention is diverted toward positive activities. Once the child is cognitively engaged, the clinician or therapist can complete the procedure. These strategies are quite similar to hypnosis and rely on the child's ability to engage in fantasy. Central to this process is the therapist's skill at engaging the child. Fortunately, the therapist's task can be relatively easy as children are generally less reality bound and more open to fantasy than are adults. It is fairly easy for many parents to learn to divert their children's attention from frightening or painful stimuli. This is done by providing the parent with basic education on behavioral principles and then coaching the parent while he or she practices the techniques during an actual painful medical procedure.

Techniques involving fantasy and attentional distraction can be used to reduce the pain of invasive procedures and the nausea and vomiting associated with chemotherapy. We (Redd et al. 1987) explored the possibility that distraction with video games could be used to block anticipatory nausea. Fifteen pediatric cancer patients with anticipatory nausea and vomiting were studied. After a no-video-game baseline assessment, all participants played commercially available video games at bedside for 10 minutes, followed immediately by a 10-minute no-video-game period, and then by a second 10-minute video game period. Results indicated that the introduction and withdrawal of the opportunity to play video games resulted in significant changes (reductions and exacerbations, respectively) in the intensity of anticipatory nausea. The effects of playing video games on anxiety were less clear-cut. Although changes in self-reported anxiety mirrored changes in anticipatory nausea, no comparisons of changes in anxiety between adjacent periods reached significance. Pulse rate and systolic-diastolic blood pressure were not consistently altered by the presentation or withdrawal of video games. In the one instance in which a physiological measure did change significantly, video game playing was associated with an increase (rather than a decrease) in systolic blood pressure. These results suggest that reductions in behavioral symptoms can be achieved independent of physiological relaxation and anxiety reduction.

Emotive Imagery

In cases of extreme, phobic-like anxiety, an individualized intervention is often required. Emotive imagery has gained wide use (Lazarus and Abramowitz 1962). Similar to distraction and hypnosis, emotive imagery takes advantage of the child's receptiveness to fantasy and involves gradual desensitization. The therapist begins working with the child in his or her office, away from the medical treatment area (Jay et al. 1985). After establishing rapport with the child, the therapist determines the child's favorite storybook hero and the things the child likes to do. The therapist then tells the child a series of stories involving the child and his or her hero. Each subsequent story brings the child closer to the feared setting, while the hero helps the child master the situation. This procedure is similar to systematic desensitization procedures used to treat phobias in adults (Wolpe 1982). The rationale is that if strong anxiety-inhibiting emotive images are elicited in the context of feared stimuli, the anxiety reaction to those stimuli will be reduced. By being told a story that involves favorite storybook heroes interacting with the phobic stimulus, the child comes to associate these stimuli with positive feelings of self-assertion, pride, and affection. As the therapist relates the story the feared stimuli are introduced in a hierarchical fashion, from least to most distressing.

As in systematic desensitization, if the child displays clear-cut anxiety, the therapist slows the story and approaches the feared object (task) less directly. Throughout the intervention the therapist is careful to be sensitive to the child's emotional reaction and is ready to pace the story according to the child's needs.

In a case reported by Diener (1984) involving a 7-year-old boy who was afraid of needles, the child was induced into a relaxation state and given an imaginary protective glove to wear before venipuncture. He became quite excited about the possibility of using the imaginary glove and complied with the therapist's instructions. During subsequent treatments the child's parents learned how to help and the therapist reduced her involvement. As the patient's mother stated, "It was amazing. David put on the magic glove and went through chemotherapy without any problem." His mother also recounted an interesting incident. One day David and his parents were waiting to see the doctor when they noticed another child crying and fighting, obviously afraid of the treatment he was about to receive. David leaned over and whispered to his mother, "Mom, should I lend him my magic glove?"

Our clinical experience is that emotive imagery can help reduce anxiety in pediatric oncology patients. However, it is important to point out that such desensitization is best used with fears that are irrational and not directly linked to aversive treatment (e.g., fears of the dark and fears of being alone). When fears are related to painful procedures (e.g., bone marrow aspiration), one would not expect emotive imagery used alone to be effective. The problem is that, after the child was desensitized, he or she would again experience the pain and aversive stimulation caused by the procedure and his or her fear would return, that is, the child would be *reconditioned*. Thus instead of a desensitization technique (i.e., emotive imagery), one would be advised to use relaxation and distraction techniques. Rather than trying to remove the fear and later to have it reestablished, the therapist devises a means of blocking the patient's perception of the pain during the actual treatment. Such a strategy would help reduce the subjective aversiveness of treatment as well as foster the reduction of anticipatory anxiety.

Hypnosis

Although the use of hypnosis to relieve acute pain has a long history, many practicing clinicians do not understand its use. In fact, many fear it (Hendler and Redd 1986). This attitude is quite unfortunate because research has demonstrated the effectiveness of hypnosis with particular pediatric patients (Hilgard and LeBaron 1984; Zeltzer et al. 1984). In the context of pediatric pain control, hypnosis involves a relatively simple dissociation process in which the patient learns to focus his or her attention to other stimuli, images, and/or thoughts that are unrelated to the source of pain. Hilgard and LeBaron (1984) coined the term *imaginative involvement* to refer to the process by which the individual becomes "hypnotized." They have maintained that this process involves the individual's becoming cognitively engaged in a task such that other stimuli are blocked or reduced in intensity.

This dissociation is common in everyday life: reading a book and being unaware of what's happening around you; playing a game of tennis and not being aware of a cut finger until after the match is over. Indeed, we (Redd et al. 1987) have argued that such imaginative involvement is exactly what is operating to produce behavioral symptom control. In clinical settings, hypnosis involves a therapist's gaining the patient's cooperation and then directing the patient's attention to images that are distinct from those associated with the treatment setting. As with other procedures, the aim is to distract the patient. Hypnosis is set apart from other methods of distraction in that the practitioner might use suggestion as a technique to induce emotional or cognitive states such as relaxation, fantasy, or positive expectations. Although all individuals are capable of this type of cognitive dissociation, some individuals are more skilled than others (Hilgard and LeBaron 1984). The essential characteristic appears to be an ability to engage in fantasy; individuals who score high on hypnotizability scales also report being able to become deeply involved in reading, in dreams, and in the aesthetic appreciation of nature. Research has shown that, as a group, children are more hypnotizable than adults (Hilgard and LeBaron 1984). They appear to be less reality bound and easily become absorbed in fantasy.

Comprehensive Behavior Modification

Comprehensive behavioral intervention packages such as those devised by Jay et al. (1985) and by Manne et al. (1990) integrate the techniques outlined above and pain and anxiety reduction procedures devised for pediatric dental patients. Treatment components may include 1) breathing exercises, 2) attentional distraction, 3) reinforcement, 4) imagery, 5) behavioral rehearsal, or 6) filmed modeling. A multifaceted program is offered to ensure maximum flexibility and to meet the particular needs of each child. With each individual child, emphasis can be placed on particular components, or the components can be adjusted to permit better tailoring of the intervention to the child's individual needs. A treatment outcome study (Jay 1988) with 56 pediatric cancer patients indicated that the intervention package yielded clinically significant reductions ($P<.01$) in children's behavioral distress, pulse rates, and self-reported pain during bone marrow aspirations.

Although the actual intervention is carried out during regularly scheduled medical procedures, the therapist or nurse meets with the patient and his or her parent during specially scheduled training sessions. The intervention represents a combination of patient education and direct behavioral treatment.

Breathing exercises. To help reduce physiological arousal and facilitate attentional distraction, deep breathing exercises are taught during training sessions and then carried out during scheduled treatments. The child might be asked to imagine blowing up a plastic bubble, taking deep breaths, and then slowly letting the air out. The therapist might explicitly pace the child's breathing by counting and squeezing his or her hand in rhythm with slow breathing. If the child shows signs of "losing it," the therapist might tell the child: "Keep it up. Slow, easy, soft breathing. You can do it, slow. Easy, . . . one, two, . . . slow, . . . three. . . . " In many ways the therapist functions as a coach. Here the therapist uses all of his or her clinical skill; the therapist must be sensitive to subtle signs of mounting anxiety in the child and, at the same time, be able to engage the child and maintain his or her attention.

Attentional distraction. To redirect attention from features in the medical environment that have come to elicit conditioned anxiety reactions (Katz et al. 1980) or conditioned nausea and/or vomiting reactions (Dolgin et al. 1985), the child can become involved in fantasy play, story telling, video games (Redd et al. 1987), or tasks in which the child can become actively absorbed. In a recent study (Manne et al. 1990), children (ages 3 to 8 years) receiving venipuncture for cancer treatment were instructed to breathe into a party blower during intravenous insertion. Blowing on the blower successfully provided an elegant form of distraction in that the child, nurse, and parent could visually verify that the child was engaging in a task that was by its nature mutually exclusive of distress behavior. Not only does the act of breathing into the blower distract the child, but also the instructions to breathe and watching the blower unravel command the child's attention. Children instructed in this technique demonstrated significantly less observable distress ($P<.01$) than those in a control group receiving comparable attention but no instruction to distract (Manne et al. 1990).

Reinforcement. Before each treatment the child and therapist decide on a toy or prize that the child will work for. Manne et al. (1990) suggested giving the patient colorful stickers for doing well. To obtain the stickers, the child's job was to keep his or her arm still for venipuncture and do the breathing exercises. We have used coloring books, small puzzles, and special outings with parents as rewards. We try to individualize the reinforcement system as much as possible. It is important to point out that the criterion for winning is not mastery of the procedure without crying or getting upset; rather, cooperation and using the skills that have been taught is all that is required. It is our experience that setting standards at realistic levels often helps turn things around for the child. By earning the prize the child starts to identify himself or herself with winning and being brave and strong. It also helps the child approach the next treatment with a more positive expectation. It is also our experience that most children want to do well and are ashamed when they resist or fight. By offering techniques that help the child tolerate procedures and specifying what behaviors are demanded of the child, the therapist provides a form of limit setting. Supplying this type of structure makes treatment less aversive and helps the child feel better about himself or herself.

Imagery.   To help distract the child's attention, the therapist uses emotive imagery during separate training sessions, as well as during scheduled treatments. The following quotation is taken from a case report provided by Jay et al. (1985) involving a young girl undergoing bone marrow aspiration:

> Pretend that Wonderwoman has come to your house and told you that she wants you to be the newest member of her Superpower Team. Wonderwoman has given you special powers. These special powers make you very strong and tough so that you can stand almost anything. She asks you to take some tests to try out these superpowers. The tests are called bone marrow aspirations and spinal taps. These tests hurt, but with your new superpowers, you can take deep breaths and lie very still. Wonderwoman will be very proud when she finds out that your superpowers work and you will be the newest member of her Superpower Team. (p. 519)

During the medical procedure, children were reminded of the imagery scenario that had been developed and were coached to use the imagery (e.g., "Remember Wonderwoman. What would she do right now?"). The emotive images presumably transform the meaning of the pain for the child and elicit motivations related to mastery over pain rather than avoidance (Zeltzer et al. 1984).

Behavioral rehearsal. To teach the child how to cooperate and to reduce anxiety arising out of fear of the unknown, the patient is taken through all phases of the procedure during training sessions. During these practice sessions the child assumes each role: playing the doctor, nurse, and patient. With a doll, the child carries out each aspect of the medical treatment that the oncologist uses during treatment. The child also practices giving proper instructions, breathing exercises, and emotive imagery material. Finally, the child takes on the role as patient and is coached to lie still and complete breathing exercises.

Filmed modeling. To further motivate children to participate in behavioral interventions, Jay (see Jay et al. 1987) has made two films portraying children in the completion of bone marrow aspiration (one for children under 8 years of age, the other for children over 8). In these films, children of approximately the same age as a patient viewing the film narrate scenes showing them going through the procedure. The patients describes their anxieties and concerns as the nurse prepares them. They also explain how they cope. The children's descriptions are realistic; they readily admit that they are afraid and that it is not easy. In her accounts of the behavioral intervention she and her colleagues have devised, Jay (see Jay et al. 1987) has stressed that the film is based on a "coping" rather than on a mastery model, that is, the film facilitates the child's identifying with the models and is more effective in reducing anxiety. Although the children depicted in the films are successful and cooperate without resistance, their anxiety is acknowledged and their hardiness is reinforced.

Clinical Issues

Behavioral intervention in pediatric oncology is typically offered as an adjunct to more traditional methods of psychosocial intervention. Children seen because of behavioral problems are also followed throughout their treatment by a clinical social worker, and their parents frequently attend parent group meetings. During the course of behavioral intervention, the behavioral clinician often addresses nonbehavioral issues. Indeed, some authors (e.g., Bandura 1962) have even argued that behavioral intervention is one of the most effective ways of building rapport and serves to facilitate work in other areas. Behavioral intervention is straightforward and does not question more sensitive issues that the patient and his or her family might wish to keep private. Thus, the patient and/or family are able to get to know the clinician in a nonthreatening context. Other issues naturally arise, and the patient is free to pursue them as he or she wishes.

Behavioral intervention is directed by three general guidelines. The first is detailed, ongoing assessment. Before beginning behavioral intervention, it is important that the clinician determine the strengths and weaknesses the child brings to treatment. The clinician must first know what the child is capable of doing. It is also important to determine at the outset the factors that contribute to the behavioral problems. Although this may be difficult and the clinician can never be sure that the assessment is complete, it is essential that the clinician understands the context in which the problem occurs. Questions the clinician might ask include: Does the child have difficulties in other areas of life? If so, what are they? When did the problems first occur and in what situation? The goal is to determine the factors that might be changed to alleviate the problem. This assessment and careful monitoring of the child's behavior continues throughout treatment. In essence, this assessment is the clinician's primary source of feedback as to how the intervention is affecting the child's behavior.

Central to behavioral assessment is clinical sensitivity. Here is when behavioral intervention resembles "art." The clinician must be sensitive to subtle changes in the patient's behavior in order to ascertain whether the patient understands, agrees, and is affected by what is being done. For example, when using imagery, distraction, and relaxation procedures, it is crucial that the clinician be aware of the patient's level of anxiety. This information allows the clinician to pace his or her work appropriately and to provide appropriate supports and prompts. In the role of coach, the skilled clinician must be exquisitely sensitive to nonverbal cues from the patient. It is important that the clinician be able to perceive subtle signs of anxiety in the patient's facial expression, voice, and/or posture. When trying to control a child's distress during a painful procedure, the therapist uses such cues to know how to pace the patient's breathing, how quickly to present distracting imagery, and whether to change to another vehicle of distraction. In this regard it is important to note that, although much has been written about patients' relative hypnotizability and it is true that highly hypnotizable patients are easier to work with, a skilled clinician can help even the more reality-bound, low-hypnotizable patients. Although it may be difficult and require additional time and patience, it is not impossible. Indeed, the clinician should look on such patients as a challenge.

A second guideline is that intervention relies on the use of positive motivation and incentives and is designed so that progress is associated with success rather than failure and frustration. In all cases, intervention proceeds through small steps. The change from one step to another is, in the ideal instance, not even perceived by the patient. The clinician begins at the patient's baseline level to help ensure success. Subsequent steps build on former. Prompts, aids, and gentle directions are used so that the child can successfully complete each new task. As the child becomes more skilled, the therapist increases the difficulty of the task so that the child is "stretched," but not frustrated. In all instances the therapist makes lavish use of praise, positive attention, and support.

A third guideline of behavioral intervention is that its effectiveness is evaluated in terms of immediate behavior change in the child. If the intervention is appropriate and of real value, it should have an immediate positive impact on the child's behavior. For example, if a procedure is intended to reduce patient distress, one would expect the child's anxiety, pain, and discomfort to diminish after the intervention is implemented. If an intervention is designed to control nausea and vomiting, there should be an immediate reduction in both. In all cases, criteria are clear and straightforward.

For many people working in the area of oncology this standard represents a welcome change from more traditional psychological-psychiatric practice in which the impact of treatment is measured in subtle changes in attitudes, often over days or weeks. In this regard, the objective criterion of treatment efficacy used by behavioral clinicians is similar to that used in clinical medicine.

Summary

Behavioral intervention is a critical component to comprehensive psychosocial care of pediatric cancer patients. Although it does not presume to address all, or even the majority, of psychosocial problems facing the young cancer patient and his or her family, it does help control the severe pain, anxiety, and nausea associated with cancer and its treatment. Behavioral intervention is valuable in the pediatric medical setting because the techniques involved 1) serve clearly identifiable functions, 2) can be taught to parents and nurses, and 3) require the clinician to define the problem clearly and to evaluate the immediate success or failure of the intervention. Perhaps because their impact is immediate and often profound, those interested in providing such services can expect to be welcomed by medical staff, patients, and their families.

References

Andrykowski MA, Redd WH: Longitudinal analysis of the development of anticipatory nausea. J Consult Clin Psychol 55:36–41, 1987

Bandura A: Social learning through imitation, in Nebraska Symposium on Motivation. Edited by Jones MR, Lincoln, NE, University of Nebraska Press, 1962, pp 26–37

Bloom K: Social elicitation of infant vocal behavior. J Exp Child Psychol 20:51–58, 1975

Bloom K: Patterning of infant vocal behavior. J Exp Child Psychol 23:367–377, 1977

Burish TG, Bradley LA (eds): Coping With Chronic Disease: Research and Applications. New York, Academic Press, 1983

Cella DF, Tross S: Psychological adjustment to survival from Hodgkin's disease. J Consult Clin Psychol 54:616–622, 1986

Clarke S, Radford M: Topical anesthesia for venipuncture. Arch Dis Child 61:1132–1134, 1986

Diener C: Controlling the Behavioral Side Effects of Cancer Treatment. Urbana, IL, Norman Baxley, 1984

Dolgin MJ, Katz ER, McGinty K, et al: Anticipatory nausea and vomiting in pediatric cancer patients. Pediatrics 75:547–552, 1985

Dolgin MJ, Phipps S, Harrow MA, et al: Parental management of fear in chronically ill and healthy children. Paper presented at meeting of the Society of Behavioral Medicine, San Francisco, CA, March 1989

Freud S: An Outline of Psychoanalysis. Translated by Strachey J. New York, Norton, 1970

Gorfinkle K: Child distress during painful medical procedures. Symposium presented at the annual meeting of the Association for the Advancement of Behavior Therapy, New York, November 1988

Hendler CS, Redd WH: Fear of hypnosis: the role of labelling in patients' acceptance of behavioral interventions. Behavior Therapy 17:2–13, 1986

Hilgard JR, LeBaron S: Relief of anxiety and pain in children and adolescents with cancer: quantitative measures and clinical observations. Int J Clin Exp Hypnosis 30:417–442, 1982

Hilgard JR, LeBaron S: Hypnotherapy of Pain in Children With Cancer. Los Altos, CA, William Kaufmann, 1984

Jacobsen PB, Manne SL, Gorfinkle KS, et al: Analysis of child and parent behavior during painful medical procedures. Health Psychol 9:559–576, 1990

Jay SM: Invasive medical procedures, in Handbook of Pediatric Psychology. Edited by Routh DK. New York, Guilford, 1988, pp 401–426

Jay SM, Ozolins M, Elliott C, et al: Assessment of children's distress during painful medical procedures. Health Psychol 2:133–147, 1983

Jay SM, Elliott CM, Ozolins M, et al: Behavioral management of children's distress during painful medical procedures. Behav Res Ther 23:513–520, 1985

Jay SM, Elliott CH, Katz ER, et al: Cognitive-behavioral and pharmacological interventions for children undergoing painful medical procedures. J Consult Clin Psychol 55:860–865, 1987

Johnson R, Baldwin D: Relationship of maternal anxiety to the behavior of young children undergoing dental extraction. J Dental Res 74:801–805, 1968

Katz ER, Kellerman H, Siegel SE: Behavioral distress in children with cancer undergoing medical procedures: developmental considerations. J Consult Clin Psychol 43:356–365, 1980

Kellerman J, Zeltzer L, Ellenberg L, et al: Adolescents with cancer: hypnosis for the reduction of acute pain and anxiety associated with medical procedures. J Adolesc Health Care 4:85–90, 1983

Koocher GP, Sallan SE: Pediatric oncology, in Psychological Management of Pediatric Problems, Vol 1. Edited by Magrab P. Baltimore, MD, University Press, 1978, pp 283–307

Kuttner L, Bowman M, Teasdale M: Psychological treatment of distress, pain, and anxiety for young children with cancer. Developmental and Behavioral Pediatrics 9:374–381, 1988

Lazarus AA, Abramowitz A: The use of "emotive imagery" in the treatment of children's phobias. Journal of Mental Sciences 108:191–195, 1962

Manne SL, Redd WH, Jacobsen PB, et al: Behavioral intervention to reduce child and parent distress during venipuncture. J Consult Clin Psychol 58:565–572, 1990

McGrath PJ, Unruh AM: Pain in Children and Adolescents. Amsterdam, Elsevier, 1987

Mechanic DK: Development of psychological distress among young adults. Arch Gen Psychiatry 36:1233–1239, 1979

Perrin E, Gerrity S: There's a demon in your belly: children's understanding of illness. Pediatrics 67:841–849, 1981

Piaget J: The Origins of Intelligence in Children. New York, Norton, 1963

Piaget J: The Psychology of the Child. New York, Basic Books, 1969

Redd WH, Andrykowski MA: Behavioral intervention in cancer treatment: controlling aversion reactions to chemotherapy. J Consult Clin Psychol 50:1018–1029, 1982

Redd WH, Andresen GV, Minagawa KY: Control of anticipatory nausea in patients undergoing cancer chemotherapy. J Consult Clin Psychol 50:14–19, 1982

Redd WH, Jacobsen PB, Die-Trill M, et al: Cognitive/attentional distraction in the control of conditioned nausea in pediatric cancer patients receiving chemotherapy. J Consult Clin Psychol 55:391–395, 1987

Reeves JL, Redd WH, Storm FK, et al: Hypnosis in the control of pain during hyperthermia treatment of cancer, in Advances in Pain Research and Therapy. Edited by Bonica JJ, Lindbland V, Iggo A. New York, Raven, 1983, pp 857–861

Ross DM, Ross SA: Childhood Pain: Current Issues, Research and Management. Baltimore, MD, Urban & Schwartzberg, 1988

Spinetta JJ, Maloney J: Death anxiety in the outpatient leukemic child. Pediatrics 56:1034–1037, 1975

van Komen R, Redd WH: Personality factors associated with anticipatory nausea/vomiting in patients receiving cancer chemotherapy. Health Psychol 4:189–202, 1985

Wahlstedt C, Kohlberg H, Moller C: Lignocaine-prilocaine cream reduces venipuncture pain (letter). Lancet 2:106, 1986

Wolpe J: The Practice of Behavior Therapy. New York, Pergamon, 1982

Wright G, Alpern G: Variables influencing children's cooperative behavior at the first dental visit. Journal of Dentistry for Children 38:124–128, 1981

Zeltzer L, LeBaron S, Zeltzer PM: The effectiveness of behavioral intervention for reduction of nausea and vomiting in children and adolescents receiving chemotherapy. J Clin Oncol 2:683–690, 1984

Chapter 7

Relaxation and Imagery for Symptom Control in Cancer Patients

Sharon A. Horowitz, A.C.S.W.
William Breitbart, M.D.

*B*ehavioral interventions are useful in the management of a wide range of symptoms encountered by cancer patients during the course of cancer illness or treatment (Table 7–1). Relaxation, distraction, and guided imagery techniques have been successfully applied, as part of a comprehensive multimodal approach, to the treatment of anxiety, pain, insomnia, anticipatory nausea and vomiting (ANV), and eating disorders in the oncology setting (Burish et al. 1987; Campbell et al. 1984; Cannici et al. 1983; Dixon 1984; Holland et al. 1991; Jay et al. 1986; Morrow and Morrel 1982; Redd 1980; Redd et al. 1982a, 1982b; Spiegel and Bloom 1983; West and Piccionne 1982). Most clinicians who work with cancer patients are now aware of the benefits of relaxation and imagery but may be unfamiliar with the specific practical techniques as they are applied in the clinical setting. We have designed this chapter to serve as a guide for the novice "relaxation" therapist. Scripts for generic relaxation and imagery exercises are illustrated with the understanding that they be modified according to the individual needs of the patient and clinician. In addition, we discuss the rationale for use of these techniques, guidelines for patient selection, and methods for overcoming common barriers to treatment.

Behavioral Interventions: Rationale and Benefits

Behavioral interventions that are useful in the cancer setting include cognitive-behavioral techniques (Table 7–2) ranging from preparatory information and self-monitoring to systematic desensitization and methods of distraction and relaxation (Breitbart and Holland 1988). Although some techniques are primarily cognitive in nature, focusing on perceptions and thought processes, other techniques are directed at modulating patterns of behavior in an effort to improve coping and relieve symptoms. Most often, techniques such as hypnosis, biofeedback, or systematic desensitization use both cognitive and behavioral elements such as muscular relaxation and cognitive distraction. Relaxation and distraction are perhaps the two most important and basic aspects of commonly used behavioral interventions with cancer patients (Mastrovito 1989).

The stimulus-response paradigm in Figure 7–1 is used to illustrate the development of behavioral symptoms and can be used as a model for behavioral intervention. In the case of Pavlov's dog, the sound of a bell (stimulus) becomes associated with the delivery of food and so results in salivation (response). In the cancer setting, the analogous conditioned paradigm could be the smell of the chemotherapy area

Table 7–1.   Behavioral applications in psychooncology

Cancer prevention
Health risk behaviors
Smoking cessation
Alcohol
Obesity
Adverse reactions to cancer treatment or diagnostic procedures
Anticipatory nausea and vomiting
Anticipatory anxiety
Phobic reactions to needles
Phobic reactions to magnetic resonance imaging
Noncompliance
Cancer-related symptoms
Cancer pain
Insomnia
Reactive anxiety and depression
Anorexia
Sexual dysfunction
Distress behavior and regression

(stimulus) and subsequent ANV (response). Relaxation is useful as an intervention for behavioral (conditioned) symptoms because it can produce an incompatible response in the setting of the conditioned stimulus (i.e., pleasant relaxation instead of tension, anxiety, or nausea). Distraction or imagery techniques are useful interventions because they allow one to alter the conditioned stimulus by manipulating perception and altering the focus of attention. Techniques such as systematic desensitization and "time-outs" are useful in extinguishing or weakening the association between stimulus and response. Relaxation techniques produce a state of calm that is incompatible with the more typical response of anxiety or distress. In the clinical setting, it is common practice to use combinations of behavioral interventions. A psychoeducational intervention is often combined with the teaching of a relaxation technique and is followed by an imagery exercise that deepens relaxation and adds the element of distraction.

Cancer patients are highly motivated to learn and practice these methods because they are often effective not only in symptom control, but also in restoring a sense of self-control, personal efficacy, and active participation in their care. Some practitioners have advocated the use of relaxation and guided imagery in cancer patients not only as a tool for promoting self-control and symptom relief, but also as a means

Table 7–2. Cognitive-behavioral techniques used by cancer patients

Cognitive	Behavioral
Preparatory information	Self-monitoring
Cognitive restructuring	Graded task management
	Systematic desensitization
Focusing	Contingency management
Controlled mental imagery	Modeling
	Behavioral rehearsal
Distraction	Relaxation
Controlled attention	Passive
Mental, behavioral	Progressive muscle
Music therapy	Music-meditation
Hypnosis	Hypnosis
Biofeedback	Biofeedback

to control tumor growth. Simonton et al. (1980) have promoted the use of relaxation and guided imagery in which the imagery used involves visualizing the body's own defenses fighting cancer cells. Cure of cancer is never a stated goal of our clinical use of cognitive-behavioral interventions. Our exclusive aim is the amelioration of behavioral symptoms in cancer patients and the improvement of quality of life. We do not generally discourage cancer patients from using these techniques to help fight their cancer; however, we are clear that there is no compelling scientific evidence that any specific visualization technique has antineoplastic effects. Aside from this controversial application of relaxation and imagery techniques, the benefits of their use in symptom control are clear.

Optimal use of cognitive-behavioral interventions for symptom control in cancer patients requires a comprehensive multimodal approach that incorporates appropriate medical assessment and intervention. Lack of side effects makes behavioral interventions quite attractive to patients who are already on multiple medications and want to avoid additional pharmacotherapy for symptoms such as insomnia or anxiety. For pain and other symptoms such as nausea and vomiting or severe anxiety, behavioral interventions are more appropriately adjunctive therapies used in combination with pharmacotherapy. Relaxation and imagery techniques are also helpful for family members of cancer patients. It is useful to teach family members these techniques not only so they can reinforce their use by patients at home and act as coaches, but also so they can reduce their own levels of distress. The use of these techniques can facilitate patient and family communication, while increasing family participation in patient care.

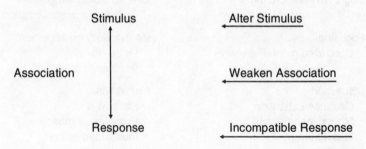

Figure 7-1.   Model for behavioral intervention

Patient Selection

Behavioral symptoms (learned or conditioned responses) commonly occur as a consequence of cancer treatment and diagnostic procedures. Almost all cancer patients with behavioral symptoms are candidates for cognitive-behavioral interventions such as relaxation and imagery. Because these techniques often involve the manipulation of concentration, attention, and perception, patients with confusional states have limited capacity to learn or practice these exercises. Occasionally these techniques can be modified so as to include even patients with mild cognitive impairment. This modification often involves the therapist's taking a more active role by orienting the patient, creating a safe and secure environment, and evoking a conditioned response to the therapist's voice or presence.

Barriers to Engaging Patients

Barriers to engaging patients in behavior therapy can be divided into therapist-based barriers and patient-based barriers. The psychiatrist who works in the cancer setting may have particular difficulty in becoming comfortable with the use of behavioral therapies. Psychiatrists are often not trained in behavioral approaches and begin work in a medical setting with a psychodynamic or psychobiological theoretical framework as opposed to a behavioral one. Behavioral therapy is often aggressive and highly directive as opposed to the more neutral approach taught most psychiatrists. Pharmacotherapy is highly effective in the management of many behavioral symptoms and seems simpler and easier to use by psychiatrists than do the labor-intensive and time-consuming nonpharmacological interventions. Perhaps most discouraging to psychiatrists interested in behavior therapy is that psychologists, social workers, and nurses (all of whom cannot prescribe medications at this time) have already established a niche for themselves as the deliverers of behavioral interventions in medical settings such as the cancer clinic or hospital. It is imperative that psychiatrists who provide consultations to cancer patients with behavioral symptoms at least be aware of the effective nonpharmacological interventions available and be able to choose wisely among practitioners who can provide such interventions. Those who choose to learn and put into practice such behavioral techniques will confront common concerns such as: "What if the patient laughs or doesn't buy it?" or "It seems too theatrical, unscientific, nonmedical; too New Age!" Overcoming such obstacles will be greatly rewarded.

Patients may have similar concerns and questions about behavioral therapies. Some may ask, "How can breathing take away my pain?" They may be frightened by the word "hypnosis" and all its connotations. Hypnosis, as patients conceptualize it, is often associated with powerful and magical properties; however, some patients become frightened at the prospect of losing control or being under the influence of someone else. We generally attempt to introduce behavioral interventions only after we have been able to establish some rapport with patients and engage them in an alliance with us. This alliance is generated around and directed toward the amelioration of a symptom that a behavioral technique may be able to help with. When introducing a specific intervention it is sometimes useful to suggest to patients, "Let's just try it and see what happens." Most patients will humor you. Occasionally, some patients may benefit from a discussion of the theoretical basis of these interventions; however, we stress that it is not important to understand why a technique works, but rather to use the technique that works. Apprehensions must be affirmed and dealt with. Patients must also feel in control of the process at all times and be reassured that they can stop at any time.

General Instructions

A general approach to using behavioral interventions in the cancer setting involves three considerations: 1) assessment of the symptom, 2) choosing a behavioral strategy, and 3) preparing the patient and the setting.

The main purpose of conducting an assessment of a conditioned or behavioral symptom is to determine what, if any, behavioral interventions are indicated (Loscalzo and Jacobsen 1990). The clinician must initially engage the patient and establish a therapeutic alliance. A history of the symptom must be taken. The clinician should review previous efforts to treat the patient's symptom and collect data regarding the nature of the symptom and its impact on the patient and his or her family.

The assessment process will lead to a variety of potential behavioral interventions. Choosing the appropriate behavioral strategy involves taking into consideration the patient's medical condition, physical and cognitive limitations, and issues such as time constraints and practical matters. For example, a patient who becomes claustrophobic while undergoing a magnetic resonance imaging (MRI) scan might best be managed with pharmacotherapy because an immediate intervention is required, and there is limited time in which to learn a relaxation technique. Also, patients with cognitive impairment or delirium will probably be unable to keep a pain diary or employ techniques that involve cognitive manipulation.

The clinician must be creative in the medical setting to establish an environment conducive to relaxation. Particularly in the hospital, the therapist must incorporate into the work interruptions such as overhead announcements, telephones ringing, and beepers going off. Although optimal conditions for relaxation are usually thought of as a quiet place without noise or interruptions, such a setting is often not available. This is not always a disadvantage because patients will be using these techniques in settings in which distractions and interruptions are commonplace, such as the chemotherapy area. It is our common practice to tape-record initial sessions with patients so that they may have an audiotape of the behavioral exercise that has been developed for them. These tapes are useful to patients as practice guides at home and can be used during episodes of distress, anxiety, pain, or insomnia. Ultimately our goal is to have patients learn relaxation and imagery exercises well enough that they can eliminate the aid of the audiotape. This is not always possible or always a necessity however. Many patients continue to rely on their audiotape with great efficacy and benefit.

Relaxation Techniques

Muscular tension, autonomic arousal, and mental distress can exacerbate anxiety, pain, and a variety of symptoms experienced by cancer patients. Therefore, interventions that reduce tension and promote a state of mental and physical relaxation can be very useful. Relaxation techniques enable cancer patients to reassert a degree of control over physiological and emotional reactions to cancer and cancer treatments. Some specific relaxation techniques include 1) passive relaxation or focused breathing, 2) passive muscle relaxation, 3) progressive muscle relaxation, 4) biofeedback, 5) hypnosis, 6) meditation, and 7) music therapy. Clinically, relaxation techniques are most helpful when combined with some imagery that allows for deeper relaxation and distraction. The use of distracting imagery often involves control over the focus of one's attention.

Passive relaxation, focused breathing, and passive muscle relaxation exercises involve focusing attention systematically on breathing, on sensations of warmth and relaxation, or on release of muscular tension in various body parts. Verbal suggestions and imagery are used to help promote relaxation. Muscle relaxation is an important component of the relaxation response and can augment the benefits of simple focused breathing exercises, leading to a deeper experience of relaxation and self-control.

Progressive or active muscle relaxation involves the active tensing and relaxing of various muscle groups in the body, focusing attention on the sensations of tension and relaxation. Clinically, in the hospital setting, relaxation is most commonly achieved through the use of a combination of focused breathing and progressive muscle relaxation exercises. Once patients are in a relaxed state, imagery techniques can then be used to induce deeper relaxation and facilitate distraction from or manipulation of a variety of cancer-related symptoms.

Script for Passive Relaxation (Focused Breathing)

The following script is a generic relaxation exercise, using passive relaxation or focused breathing, that is based on and integrates the work of Erickson (1959), Benson (1975), and others (Loscalzo and Jacobsen 1990).

Why don't you begin by finding a comfortable position. [It could be in a bed or in a chair.] Slowly allow your body to unwind and just let it go. That's it . . . I wonder if you can allow your body to become as calm as possible . . . just let it go, just let your body sink into that bed [or chair] . . . feel free to move or shift around in any way that your body needs to, to find that comfortable position. You need not try very hard, simply and easily allow yourself to follow the sound of my voice as you allow your body to find itself a safe, comfortable position to relax in.

If you like, [patient's name], you can gently allow your eyes to close, just let the lids cover your eyes . . . allow your eyes to sink back deeply into their sockets . . . that's it, just let them go, falling back gently and deeply into their sockets as your lids begin to feel heavier and heavier. As you allow your head to fall back deeply into the pillow, feeling the weight of your head sinking into the pillow as you breath out, just breath out, one big breath. Slowly, if you can begin to turn your attention to your breathing. Notice your breath for a few moments, how much air you take in, how much air you let out, and just breath evenly and naturally, and with the sound of my voice I wonder if you can begin to take in more air, breathing in and out, in and out, that's it, gradually breathing in and out . . . in and out . . . breathing in calmness and quietness, breathing out tiredness and frustration, that's it . . . let it go, it's not important to you now . . . breathing in quietness and control, breathing out fear and tension . . . breathing in and out . . . . in and out . . . you can enjoy breathing in this relaxed way for as long as you need to. You are peaceful now as you continue to observe your even and steady breathing that is allowing you to feel gentle and calm, breathing that is allowing you to feel a gentle calm, that's it, breathing relaxation in and tension out . . . in and out . . . breathing in quietness and control, breathing out tiredness and tension . . . that's it [patient's name] as you continue to notice the quietness and stillness of your body. Why don't you take a few quiet moments to experience this process more fully.

It may be helpful for the clinician to mark the end of an exercise by increasing the pace, raising the volume of voice, and shifting position. Additionally it is helpful for the clinician to both pace and model for the patient. This includes positioning yourself as similarly to the patient as possible (e.g., closing eyes, assuming a position of relaxation, and breathing at the same rate). If the patient exhibits any visible anxiety or agitation, this can be briefly explored verbally, and then, if appropriate, the exercise can be continued.

Script for Passive Muscle Relaxation

The clinician requests that the patient find a comfortable position, either sitting or lying down and then may state:

Gradually allow your body to lie still . . . you may move around and adjust your body in any way that you like until your body finds itself in a comfortable position. Gently allow your eyes to close and allow your mind to focus inwards, gradually becoming aware of how your body feels. Just continue breathing normally . . . breathing in and out . . . in and out . . . breathing in quietness and relaxation . . . breathing out tiredness and tension, breathing it right out of you. Now, I wonder if you can do a mental scan of your body. Notice how it feels. Are there any parts that are more relaxed than others? Any parts that feel more tight or tense than others? Any parts that need special attention? As you slowly begin to focus your thoughts inwards, tuning out any outside noises or distractions, they are not important to you now. Simply and easily allow your body to sink deeper and deeper into your bed. . . .

The clinician requests that the patient mentally begin to scan the entire body, focusing on individual body parts in a progressive manner including the feet, legs, thighs, buttocks, pelvis, stomach, chest, arms, shoulders, and back. The head and facial muscles are also scanned and particular attention can be paid to individual facial features such as the jaw, forehead, eyes, and neck because a considerable amount of tension can be stored in these areas. The exercise can begin with relaxation of muscles either in the head and face or in the feet and legs, and proceed naturally up or down the body. Occasionally a painful part of the body may need more attention or may need to be avoided, depending on the patient's comfort.

Imagery may also be incorporated into the relaxation technique by suggesting that the patient imagine the tension draining or flowing out of a particular body part or by suggesting that the patient imagine healing, soothing air circulating around specific areas:

> Imagine this healing, soothing air dancing around each individual toe, that's it . . . bathing each toe with soft, gentle air as you feel each toe becoming lighter and softer, lighter and softer . . . that's it, as you allow all the tension and tightness to float away . . . just float away, as you feel yourself becoming more and more relaxed . . . and slowly, imagine this air traveling from your toes to your feet, washing over your feet as they begin to sink deeper and deeper into the bed . . . just let them go, that's it . . . as your feet begin to feel heavier and heavier, as all the tension and tightness floats away. . . .

Script for Active or Progressive Muscle Relaxation

This exercise involves the patient actively tensing and then relaxing specific body parts. Once again, it may be helpful if the clinician paces and models for the patient.

> Now, I wonder if you can tense up every muscle in your body . . . that's it, squeeze in the muscles . . . hold it, and then just let it go . . . once more, tense up your muscles . . . make them very tight and tense, hold

it, hold it . . . and then breath out, and let your muscles relax, just let them go. . . . Now, as your body begins to feel more and more relaxed, clench your jaw, squeeze it tight, clench it and then let it go . . . now open your mouth wide, as wide as it will go, stick out your tongue, stick it way out, hold it and then let it go. Feel your head becoming more and more relaxed, as it sinks down into the pillow, allowing all the tension and tightness to drift out of it . . . Now, I wonder if you can lift up your shoulders, lift them up, up to your ears, hold them there, squeezing them tightly, squeeze, and then let them drop down, just let them go . . . and then once more lift them up . . . hold it . . . then let them go . . . as you feel all the tightness and tension in your shoulders begin to drain away. . . . Now, I wonder if you can clench your hands into a fist, make a tight fist as your whole arm tightens, tense your arms as you squeeze in your fingers tighter and tighter . . . and now just let them go, once more now make a fist, a tight fist, hold it, and then let it go.

As with passive muscle relaxation, the clinician guides the patient through the exercise, requesting the patient to tense and release specific muscles in a progressive order.

Imagery Techniques

Imagery—the use of one's imagination—is another technique that is effective in further facilitating and deepening relaxation as well as adding the important component of distraction to symptom control interventions. Imagery is usually used in conjunction with other exercises such as focused breathing and passive or progressive muscle relaxation. Imagery (often referred to as "guided imagery") is most effective when the specific image is obtained from the patient. The clinician may ask the patient to close his or her eyes and think of a place, an activity, or an experience in which the patient felt most safe and secure. The clinician may provide suggestions for the patient such as a favorite beach scene, a room in a house, or riding a bicycle in a state park. Once the patient identifies the scene, the clinician may ask the patient to elaborate on the scene, asking for specific details such as the temperature, season, time of day, type of ocean (calm or with big waves), and so on. The clinician then uses this information and describes an image for the patient in detail.

The skill is for the clinician to be as flexible and as creative as possible and to elaborate on the scene, using all aspects of the senses and bodily sensations such as "feel the suns rays touch your skin, allow your skin to feel warm and tingly all over" or "breath in the fresh, clear air, allow it to fill your lungs with its freshness" or "feel the fresh dew of the grass under your feet." The clinician can focus on "aromas in the garden" or the "sounds of birds singing," always reminding the patient to breath evenly and steadily as he or she feels more and more relaxed and more and more in control. If possible, the clinician should avoid volunteering an image or scene for the patient because the clinician is unaware of the association or meaning the image may have for the patient. For example, a patient may have a fear of the water, and therefore a beach scene may invoke feelings of fear and loss of control.

Script for Guided Imagery: Exercise 1

The clinician requests that the patient find a comfortable position, either sitting or lying down, and then may state:

> Once you are in a comfortable position, I wonder if you can continue lying there with your eyes closed, continuing to breath in and out . . . in and out to the sound of my voice. Let your mind wander . . . just let it go . . . and if any unwanted thoughts come into your mind, you can allow then to pass out as easily as they came in. . . . You don't need them now . . . they are not important to you now. You have the ability to control your thoughts. You have the ability to be in control.

The clinician now begins to describe a specific image in detail as originally suggested by the patient:

> Slowly, I wonder if you can allow your mind to travel . . . to travel far away to your favorite beach. The beach that you have many fond memories of. I wonder if you can imagine that it's almost the end of the day and the beach is deserted . . . and the sun, while setting, is still warm, as it beats down . . . and makes your skin feel tingly and warm all over. As you begin to walk on the sand, you can feel the granules underneath your feet. Step evenly and steadily along the sand. As you look around, you can see the different colors in the sky. You can see for miles off into the distance and you feel exhilarated and free because no one is around you. You are alone and in control.
>
> As you walk closer to the edge of the ocean the sand is becoming a little damp and you can feel the dampness underneath your feet—it

feels refreshing. As you continue walking, you may notice a few odds and ends on the sand, maybe something that the ocean brought in . . . some shells perhaps. They may be broken from being knocked against the rocks . . . or there may be a few bits of seaweed or some jellyfish. You stop to notice them as you walk past . . . marveling at the wonders of nature. As you get to the edge of the ocean, you can feel the tiny little ripples of water washing over your feet . . . bouncing over your feet making you feel light and fresh. The water is warm—it soothes your feet. Washing back and forth . . . back and forth.

As you keep walking you see your rubber raft. This is your old dependable rubber raft. You get to the raft and you secure it in your hands and lie down on it letting your whole body sink into the raft—just let it go . . . that's it. Slowly you kick off as the raft begins to take you away. The ocean is very calm and very gentle. Your whole body begins to unwind and sink deeper and deeper into the raft as you feel more and more relaxed. This raft allows you to drift off . . . and underneath you can feel the ripples of the ocean . . . rocking back and forth . . . back and forth as you continue to float away evenly and gently. You can become aware of the sun beating down on your skin. You are aware of the sounds around you—you can hear the ocean washing against the rocks as the waves rock back and forth . . . back and forth. You can hear the gulls crying in the distance. There is a very tiny protected bay that you are floating away in. It is a very calm and peaceful day, and you are feeling more and more relaxed. You are in control now . . . and as you continue to sail away, all your troubles and problems wash right out of you. They're not important to you now. You don't need them now. What's important is that your whole body, from the tip of your toes all the way up to the top of your head, is relaxed and calm in this very safe and private place that is your own. You can continue to lie here as you rock back and forth . . . back and forth for as long as you need to.

When you are ready, you can slowly readjust yourself to the sound of my voice and I am going to count slowly backwards from *10* and with each count backwards, you can become more and more familiar with where you are. Perhaps when I get to number 5 you may want to open your eyes or you can keep then closed for as long as you need to. Ten, nine . . . become aware of the sounds around you . . . eight, seven . . . become aware of the temperature of the room—how does it feel? how does your body feel? . . . six, five . . . you can open your eyes now if you want to or you can keep them closed . . . four, three, two, one. You can stay in this relaxed position for as long as you need to. When you feel ready you may slowly prepare to sit up.

Script for Guided Imagery: Exercise 2

The clinician requests that the patient find a comfortable position, or remains there if he or she has just completed a relaxation exercise, and then may state:

I wonder if you can allow your mind to travel to that garden that you know. To the garden that you have devotedly planted and created. A garden that has intricacies and uniqueness only you know. I wonder if you can imagine yourself standing in this garden. It's a warm spring day—the sun is up, it's bright and shining and you are all alone. You are in a safe and quiet place. No one can distract you.

Now, I wonder if you can allow your mind to appreciate the full beauty of this garden. The trees around you; the blue clear sky. The grass underneath your feet and the flowers that you planted. I wonder if you can imagine yourself going up to each individual flower that is now starting to blossom, that is now opening up toward the sun to drink in all the glory of the sun's rays. As you marvel at these flowers, you examine each individual petal—its color, the brightness and clearness of the colors. As you lean forward and breath in the unique aroma of each flower, each flower whether it's lavender or buttercup, marigold, rose, or bluebell has its own individual aroma that you can identify even with your eyes closed. If you breath it in, breath it into your lungs. Let your whole body fill with the pleasure. The very simple pleasure of the untainted clear aroma of the flowers that you planted.

As you carry on walking through your garden you can feel the grass underneath your feet. You can hear the birds singing. You also know each individual bird. These too you can recognize with your eyes closed just by the sounds they make. You know exactly what birds they are. Exactly what their individual habits are; their mating calls; the kinds of nests they build. Even the type of twigs or materials that they use to build their nests. You recognize each bird by its coloring. How they fly and you smile at them. These birds are very familiar to you. They're your friends. They kept you company when you built this garden from nothing. When you carefully and patiently planted the seeds of your garden and now you can fully appreciate the glory and pride of your efforts. As you continue to walk, you walk towards your fruit trees that you planted, and it's spring and the tree is bearing fruit. Your favorite fruit. Whether it be an apple, pear, or cherry. You walk up to the tree and pick the fruit. The piece of fruit is perfect and ripe and you decide to taste it. Take a big bite. You become aware of the texture and taste of the piece of fruit. You chew it slowly and swallow it. It fills your whole body with the delight and sensation of eating something that is delicious and that you too created. . . .

Application of Relaxation and Imagery to Specific Problems of Cancer Patients

Anxiety, Phobias, and Panic

The types of anxiety seen in the cancer setting include 1) reactive anxiety related to the stress of cancer illness or treatment, 2) anxiety that is a manifestation of a medical or physiological problem (organic anxiety disorder) related to cancer, and 3) phobias, panic, and chronic anxiety disorders that predate the cancer diagnosis, but are exacerbated during the course of illness.

Occasionally, patients will have their first episode of panic or phobia while in the medical setting. At Memorial Sloan-Kettering Cancer Center, approximately 20% of patients developed anxiety or claustrophobia so severe that they could not complete an MRI scan (Brennan et al. 1988). Because the presence of one of these anxiety disorders (e.g., panic attack, needle phobia, or claustrophobia) can complicate treatment, an early psychiatric consultation is recommended. The techniques available to treat these disorders include both behavioral approaches and short-term pharmacological interventions. If there is the luxury of time (days to weeks) and the patient will have to face the stressor (e.g., venipuncture and bone marrow aspiration) repeatedly, relaxation and distraction techniques can help the patient gain some control over his or her fear.

The goal of a behavioral intervention in this case is therefore to break the association between harmless signals and the anticipation of hurt and to modify the behaviors that occur in order to avoid the anticipated harm. The patient is first taught to relax with passive breathing accompanied by either passive or active muscle relaxation. Once in a relaxed state, the patient is exposed to systematically increasing successive approximations of the threatening situation and eventually to the situation itself. For example, a female patient who became diabetic refused to have insulin injections on a daily basis due to her fear of needles. She was first taught breathing exercises and then taught to pair the breathing exercise with systematic exposure (initially in her imagination and then in external reality) to an injection. Eventually, she learned to give herself the injections on a daily basis. Ideally, the clinician will have several days to teach and reinforce relaxation before the administration of the actual injection. Another patient, a 27-year-old woman, was claustrophobic and felt unable to remain motionless during an MRI. Once relaxed, she chose to imagine herself lying on a cloud on a clear, brisk day. She imagined herself floating away in the vast openness of the sky as she observed the world below her that was unable to touch her or frighten her.

Often, however, the need for procedures is too acute and we prescribe benzodiazepines (e.g., alprazolam 0.25–1.0 mg po tid) in addition to providing emotional support to help the phobic patient undergo necessary procedures. Combination drug and behavioral treatment is quite effective for patients with high levels of anxiety related to cancer. Holland et al. (1991) compared the efficacy of a behavioral intervention and a pharmacotherapy for the treatment of anxiety and distress in cancer patients. Most of the patients had a diagnosis of adjustment disorder with anxious and depressed mood. Half of the patients were taught a progressive muscle relaxation exercise that was tape-recorded and practiced three times a day. The other half were prescribed alprazolam 0.5 mg po tid. For levels of anxiety and depression that were in the mild-to-moderate range, both the behavioral and the pharmacological interventions were equally effective. It was only for patients with high levels of anxiety and depression that the pharmacological intervention proved more successful. For patients with anxiety and distress related to cancer (reactive anxiety), we typically employ combinations of such therapies in an effort to maximize symptom control. (For an extensive discussion of anxiety and depression, see Chapter 1.)

Cancer Pain

Behavioral interventions are effective in the management of acute procedure-related cancer pain (Table 7–3), and as an adjunct in the management of chronic cancer pain (Table 7–4) (Fotopoulos et al. 1979; Spiegel and Bloom 1983; Turk and Rennert 1981). Hypnosis, biofeedback, and multicomponent cognitive-behavioral interventions have been used to provide comfort and minimize pain in adults, children, and adolescents undergoing bone marrow aspirations, spinal taps, and other painful procedures (Hilgard and LeBaron 1982; Jay et al. 1986; Kellerman et al. 1983). Typically, behavioral interventions (e.g., hypnosis) used in the management of acute, procedure-related pain employ the basic elements of relaxation, distraction or diversion of attention, and altered perception of pain. (For an in-depth discussion of the use of cognitive behavioral techniques, such as hypnosis, for chronic pain related to tumor progression and impingement on pain-sensitive structures or due to some neurotoxic effect of cancer treatment, see Chapter 3.)

In chronic cancer pain, cognitive-behavioral techniques are most effective when they are employed as part of a multimodal, multidisci-

Table 7–3. Behavioral interventions: acute procedure-related cancer pain

Study	Type of pain	Intervention	Outcome
Hilgard and LeBaron 1982	Bone marrow aspiration in children	Hypnosis	Decreased pain
Jay et al. 1986	Bone marrow aspiration and lumbar puncture	Cognitive-behavioral multicomponent program[a]	Decreased pain
Kellerman et al. 1983	Bone marrow aspiration and lumbar puncture in adolescents	Hypnosis	Decreased pain
Redd et al. 1982b	Hyperthermia in adults	Hypnosis	Decreased pain
Zeltzer and LeBaron 1982	Bone marrow aspiration and lumbar puncture in adolescents	Hypnosis	Decreased pain

[a]Filmed modeling, breathing training, imagery-distraction, behavioral rehearsal, and positive reinforcement.

plinary approach (Breitbart and Holland 1990). Adequate medical assessment and management of cancer pain are essential. Mild to moderate levels of residual pain can be effectively managed with behavioral techniques that are quite similar to those used for anxiety, phobias, and ANV. Relaxation techniques are used to help the patient achieve a relaxed state. Once in a relaxed state, the cancer patient with pain can use a variety of imagery techniques including 1) pleasant distracting imagery; 2) transformational imagery, and 3) dissociative imagery (Breitbart and Holland 1990). Transformational imagery involves the imaginative transformation of either the painful sensation itself or the context of pain, or both. Patients can imaginatively transform a sensation of pain in their arm, for instance, into a sensation of warmth or cold. They can use such imagery as "dipping their arm into a bucket of cold spring water" or into a "vat of warm honey." Such techniques can also be used to alter the context of the pain. Dissociative imagery or dissociated somatization refers to the use of the imagination to disconnect or dissociate from the pain experience. Specifically, patients can sometimes imagine that they leave their pain-racked body in bed and walk about for 5 or 10 minutes pain free. Patients can also imagine that a particularly painful part of their body becomes disconnected or dissociated from the rest of them, resulting in a period of freedom from pain. These techniques can provide much needed respite from pain. Even short periods of relief from pain can break the vicious pain cycle that entraps many cancer patients.

Table 7–4.   Behavioral interventions: chronic cancer pain

Study	Intervention	Outcome
Fotopoulos et al. 1979	EMG, EEG, biofeedback	Decreased pain
Spiegel and Bloom 1983[a]	Group therapy and self-hypnosis	Decreased pain
Turk and Rennert 1981	Cognitive-behavioral multicomponent program	Decreased pain

Note.   EMG = electromyogram; EEG = electroencephalogram.
[a]Controlled study.

ANV Related to Chemotherapy

During the course of chemotherapy, many patients become sensitized to the treatment, develop phobic-like reactions, and even develop conditioned responses to stimuli in the hospital setting. As a result of being conditioned by the experience of profound nausea and vomiting secondary to highly emetic chemotherapy agents, patients report being nauseated in anticipation of treatment (see Chapter 5). A conservative estimate of the prevalence of ANV is at least 33% of patients (Morrow 1982). The factors that increase the likelihood of developing ANV are 1) severity of posttreatment nausea and vomiting (PNV) (high density, duration, and frequency), 2) a pattern of increasing nausea and vomiting, and 3) receiving highly emetic drugs (cisplatin) or combinations of chemotherapies (Jacobsen et al. 1988).

Given the relationship between intensity of PNV and the development of ANV, the efficacy of antiemetic regimens in the management of these symptoms becomes increasingly important. The most effective regimens currently combine several agents such as metoclopramide, steroids, and lorazepam. These drugs are given a few hours before chemotherapy and are continued by intravenous infusion up to 36 hours after completion of chemotherapy. Parenteral lorazepam reduces vomiting and produces a mild amnesia for the vomiting episodes. Metoclopramide is a dopamine antagonist and so can induce extrapyramidal side effects that are reversible with treatment. There is only one reported case of tardive dyskinesia secondary to intravenous metoclopramide as used in an antiemetic regimen during cancer chemotherapy (Breitbart 1986). Rapid-onset, short-acting benzodiazepines are helpful in controlling ANV once it has developed. Alprazolam has been shown to be clinically effective in reducing ANV in doses of 0.25 to 0.5 mg three to four times a day, given for 1–2 days before chemotherapy (Greenberg et al. 1987).

Behavioral control of ANV has proven to be highly effective (Redd et al 1987). The techniques that have been studied (Table 7–5) include 1) relaxation training with guided imagery, 2) video game distraction (with children), and 3) systematic desensitization. It is unclear whether muscular relaxation or cognitive-attentional distraction is the key element in the efficacy of some of these techniques. Chemotherapy nurses trained in these techniques can remarkably improve the quality of life for chemotherapy patients.

Insomnia

Behavioral interventions have been successfully applied to the treatment of insomnia in cancer patients (Table 7–6). Cannici et al. (1983) studied 15 patients with secondary insomnia due to cancer and showed a marked reduction in mean sleep onset latency after progressive muscle relaxation training. Stam et al. (1986) showed an increase in duration of sleep using relaxation and imagery techniques. Such techniques are useful nonpharmacological interventions that help keep medication use to a minimum. Occasionally sleep disturbance in cancer patients may be due to a concomitant psychiatric disorder such as depression or delirium. Obviously in these cases specific treatment for the underlying disorder is a preferred approach. Pharmacotherapy using benzodiazepines, neuroleptics, or antidepressants may also be indicated when sleep disturbance is due to medication side effects or to some other organic etiology.

Cancer Anorexia

Behavioral interventions are commonly used to treat a variety of eating disorders in cancer patients including conditioned anorexia, swallow-

Table 7–5. Behavioral interventions: anticipatory nausea and vomiting (ANV)

Controlled studies	Intervention	Outcome
Burish and Lyles 1979, 1981; Burish et al. 1987	Progressive muscle relaxation with imagery	Decreased pretreatment and posttreatment nausea Decreased anxiety Decreased ANV Prevents ANV
Morrow and Morrell 1982	Systematic desensitization	Decreased ANV
Redd et al. 1982a	Hypnosis, passive relaxation, and imagery	Decreased pretreatment and posttreatment nausea Decreased ANV
Redd et al. 1987	Cognitive-attentional distraction and video games	Decreased ANV

ing difficulties, and nausea and vomiting (Table 7–7). (For an extensive discussion of the etiology, assessment, and management of these problems, see Chapter 4.) Assessment of anorexia in the cancer setting is quite complex. Anorexia as a symptom in cancer patients often has multiple etiologies including factors related to the cancer itself, depression, and learned or conditioned elements. Dixon (1984) reported on a study of 55 nutritionally at-risk cancer patients who were randomized to four intervention groups. One group received nutritional support alone, one received relaxation training only, a third group received both supplementation and relaxation, and a fourth group was a no-intervention control group. Weight gain was greatest for the relaxation groups who were taught deep abdominal breathing, autosuggestion, progressive relaxation, and imagery. Campbell et al. (1984) showed that a relaxation and imagery exercise program was associated with weight gain and improvement in performance status. Conditioned difficulties with eating, swallowing, and nausea have been managed successfully with systematic desensitization (Redd 1980; West and Piccionne 1982). Hypnosis has been used in children with cancer, resulting in improved appetite and weight gain (LeBaw et al. 1975).

Neurologically Impaired Patients

Working with this population requires that the clinician take a more active role in the relaxation process. This involves the use of nonverbal approaches as well as direct suggestion. The clinician first orients the patient to the clinician's presence and sound of voice. The clinician may take the patient's hand and say, "Hello [patient's name], this is [clinician's name]. You are in [name of hospital], and you are safe now. When I am with you, no one is going to bother you or distract you. You and I are going to spend some quiet time together. You are in a safe and

Table 7–6. Behavioral interventions: insomnia

Study	Intervention	Outcome
Cannici et al. 1983	Progressive muscle relaxation training	Decreased sleep onset latency
Stam et al. 1986	Somatic focusing imagery training	Increased sleep duration

secure place." The clinician can repeat soothing and reassuring state-ments to the patient. Based on the patient's cognitive level of function-ing, the clinician may then begin to actively direct the patient to close his or her eyes and to participate in passive or progressive muscle relaxation. The skill of this technique requires that the clinician be as flexible and creative as possible, using all of the patient's senses (perhaps using perfume and requesting that the patient breath in the healing and soothing aroma of the perfume), as well as focusing on the patient's strengths and functioning that are not impaired. For example, a patient may be confused or expressively aphasic, but may still be able to follow directions.

Summary

Relaxation and imagery techniques have a role in the management of a wide range of symptoms in cancer patients. In this chapter, we have provided a theoretical and empirical rationale for the application of such behavioral techniques in the management of cancer-related anxi-ety, distress, pain, anorexia, insomnia, and ANV. Scripts for relaxation and imagery exercises have been provided to help encourage therapists

Table 7–7.   Behavioral interventions: cancer anorexia

Study	Intervention	Outcome
Campbell et al. 1984	Relaxation imagery	Weight gain, improved Karnofsky performance status
Dixon 1984	Relaxation, nutritional supplementation	Weight gain
LeBaw et al. 1975	Hypnosis in children	Increased appetite and weight gain
Redd 1980	Relaxation, in vivo desensitization in adults	Improved eating and swallowing
West and Piccionne 1982	Systematic desensitization	Improved eating in adults, decreased nausea and vomiting

unfamiliar with these techniques to begin practicing them with patients. (For more detailed instructions on technique and practical applications of relaxation and imagery interventions, see Berenson 1988. Other useful readings include Benson 1975, Loscalzo and Jacobsen 1990, and Mastrovito 1989.)

References

Benson H: The Relaxation Response. New York, William Morrow, 1975

Berenson S: The cancer patient, in Relaxation and Imagery: Tools for Therapeutic Communication and Intervention. Edited by Zahourek R. Philadelphia, PA, WB Saunders, 1988, pp 168–191

Breitbart W: Tardive dyskinesia associated with high dose intravenous metaclopramide (letter). N Engl J Med 315:518, 1986

Breitbart W, Holland JC: Psychiatric complications of cancer, in Current Therapy in Hematology Oncology, 3rd Edition. Edited by Brain MC, Carbone PP. Philadelphia, PA, BC Decker, 1988, pp 268–274

Breitbart W, Holland J: Psychiatric aspects of cancer pain, in Advances in Pain Research and Therapy, Vol 16. Edited by Foley K, Bonica JJ, Ventafridda V. New York, Raven, 1990, pp 73–88

Brennan SC, Redd WH, Jacobsen PB, et al: Anxiety and panic during magnetic resonance scans (letter). Lancet 2:512, 1988

Burish TG, Lyles JN: Effectiveness of relaxation training in reducing the aversiveness of chemotherapy in the treatment of cancer. J Behav Ther Exp Psychiatry 10:357–361, 1979

Burish TG, Lyles JN: Effectiveness of relaxation training in reducing adverse reactions to cancer chemotherapy. J Behav Med 4:65–78, 1981

Burish TG, Carey MP, Krozely MG, et al: Conditioned side effects induced by cancer chemotherapy: prevention through behavioral treatment. J Consult Clin Psychol 55:42–48, 1987

Campbell D, Dixon J, Sanderford L, et al: Relaxation: its effect on the nutritional status and performance status of clients with cancer. J Am Diet Assoc 84:201–204, 1984

Cannici J, Malcolm R, Peck LA: Treatment of insomnia in cancer patients using muscle relaxant training. J Behav Ther Exp Psychiatry 14:251–256, 1983

Dixon J: Effect of nursing interventions on nutritional and performance status in cancer patients. Nurs Res 33:330–335, 1984

Erickson MH: Hypnosis in painful terminal illness. Am J Clin Hypn 1:1117–1121, 1959

Fotopoulos SS, Graham C, Cook MR: Psychophysiologic control of cancer pain, in Advances in Pain Research and Therapy, Vol 2. Edited by Bonica JJ,

Ventafridda V. New York, Raven, 1979, pp 231–244

Greenberg DB, Surman OS, Clarke J, et al: Alprazolam for phobic nausea and vomiting related to cancer chemotherapy. Cancer Treatment Reports 71:549–550, 1987

Hilgard E, LeBaron S: Relief of anxiety and pain in children and adolescents with cancer: quantitative measures and clinical observations. Int J Clin Exp Hypn 30:417–442, 1982

Holland JC, Morrow G, Schmale A, et al: A randomized clinical trial of alprazolam versus progressive muscle relaxation in cancer patients with anxiety and depressive symptoms. J Clin Oncol 9:1004–1011, 1991

Jacobsen PB, Andrykowski MA, Redd WH, et al: Nonpharmacologic factors in the development of posttreatment nausea with adjuvant chemotherapy for breast cancer. Cancer 61:379–385, 1988

Jay S, Elliott C, Varni J: Acute and chronic pain in adults and children with cancer. J Consult Clin Psychol 54:601–607, 1986

Kellerman J, Zeltzer L, Ellenberg L, et al: Adolescents with cancer: hypnosis for the reduction of acute pain and anxiety associated with medical procedures. J Adolesc Health Care 4:85–90, 1983

LaBaw W, Holton C, Tewell K, et al: The use of self hypnosis by children with cancer. Am J Clin Hypn 17:233–238, 1975

Loscalzo M, Jacobsen PB: Practical behavioral approaches to the effective management of pain and distress. Journal of Psychosocial Oncology 8:139–169, 1990

Mastrovito R: Behavioral techniques: progressive relaxation and self-regulatory therapies, in Handbook of Psychooncology: Psychological Care of the Patient With Cancer. Edited by Holland JC, Rowland JH. New York, Oxford Press, 1989, pp 492–501

Morrow GR: Prevalence and correlates of anticipatory nausea and vomiting in chemotherapy patients. J Natl Cancer Inst 68:585–588, 1982

Morrow GR, Morrell BS: Behavioral treatment for the anticipatory nausea and vomiting induced by cancer chemotherapy. N Engl J Med 307:1476–1480, 1982

Redd WH: Invivo desensitization in the treatment of chronic emesis following gastrointestinal surgery. Behavior Therapy 11:421–427, 1980

Redd WH, Andresen GV, Minagawa RY: Hypnotic control of anticipatory emesis in patients receiving cancer chemotherapy. J Consult Clin Psychol 50:14–19, 1982a

Redd WB, Reeves JL, Storm JK, et al: Hypnosis in the control of pain during hyperthermia treatment of cancer, in Advances in Pain Research and Theory, Vol 5. Edited by Bonica JJ, Lindblom U, Iggo A, et al. New York, Raven, 1982b, pp 857–861

Redd WH, Jacobsen PB, Die-Trill M, et al: Cognitive/attentional distraction in the control of conditioned nausea in pediatric cancer patients receiving chemotherapy. J Consult Clin Psychol 55:391–395, 1987

Simonton OC, Matthews-Simonton S, Sparks TF: Psychological intervention in the treatment of cancer. Psychosomatics 21:226–233, 1980

Spiegel D, Bloom JR: Group therapy and hypnosis reduce metastatic breast carcinoma pain. Psychosom Med 4:333–339, 1983

Stam H, Bultz B, Pittman C: Psychosocial problems and interventions in a referred sample of cancer patients. Psychosom Med 48:539–548, 1986

Turk DC, Rennert KS: Pain and the terminally ill cancer patient: a cognitive social learning perspective, in Behavior Therapy in Terminal Care: A Humanistic Approach. Edited by Sobel H. Cambridge, MA, Ballinger, 1981, pp 15–44

West B, Piccionne C: Cognitive-behavioral techniques in treating anorexia and depression in a cancer patient. Behavioral Therapist 5:115–117, 1982

Zeltzer L, LeBaron S: Hypnosis and nonhypnotic techniques for reduction of pain and anxiety painful procedures in children and adolescents with cancer. J Pediatr 101:1032–1035, 1982

Chapter 8

Terminally Ill Cancer Patients

William Breitbart, M.D.
Jon A. Levenson, M.D.
Steven D. Passik, Ph.D.

*P*sychiatrists and psychologists who work in the oncology setting are often called on to assist in the treatment of patients in the far-advanced stages of illness. As the possibility of cure or prolongation of life becomes remote, treatment focuses on symptom control and enhancement of patients' quality of life. In this chapter, we address issues of physical and psychological symptom control crucial for the mental health professional working with terminally ill cancer patients.

It is important to address what exactly we mean by "terminally ill." The definition can differ based on setting (i.e., in the cancer center versus the hospice), discipline (i.e., an oncologist versus an internist), and individual physician or patient point of view. Lesko and Holland (1989) pointed out that patients often view themselves as being terminally ill after a serious intensification of their medical symptoms. Doctors, on the other hand, are more likely to define "terminal" on the basis of failure to respond to known curative measures. Thus patients decide that they are "terminal" based on how they feel symptomatically, whereas physicians rely on less subjective criteria. Symptoms are central to patients' sense of their future and thus to their ability to maintain hope. Therefore, the prompt recognition and effective treatment of psychiatric and physical symptoms become critically important to the well-being of patients with advanced disease.

In this chapter we use the phrases *terminally ill, terminal phases of illness,* or *advanced cancer* to refer to the condition of patients who have a life expectancy of 3–6 months and for whom care has generally switched to a palliative mode. For such patients, treatment is no longer aimed at cure but at palliation and comfort. In our specialized setting (a tertiary-care cancer center) it is not uncommon to find patients (who meet this definition of "terminal") still receiving active treatments aimed at the extension of life. Throughout this chapter, we use the term *dying* to refer solely to patients in the last days to hours of life.

Cancer patients in the terminal phases of illness are uniquely vulnerable to both physical and psychiatric complications. The high prevalence of distressing physical symptoms, such as pain, makes the assessment of psychiatric symptoms more difficult and requires that the mental health professional possess specialized knowledge and skills. Additionally, the psychiatrist treating distressed, terminally ill cancer patients must be aware of the common painful physical symptoms and take an active role in ensuring their adequate control. Left unchecked, physical and psychiatric symptoms can have a synergistic negative impact on patients' quality of life. It is with this in mind that we present a chapter dedicated to the control of both physical and psychiatric symptoms in terminally ill cancer patients.

Controlling Psychiatric Symptoms

Many terminally ill cancer patients are able to cope with advancing illness and debility without formal psychiatric intervention. For such patients, the oncologist, nurse, and social worker provide sufficient medical and psychosocial care during the terminal phase of illness, and their families provide them with a sense of being cared for, valued, and loved. Spiritual and religious counseling often plays a vital role as disease advances. Terminal illness is not a psychiatric disorder; however, terminally ill cancer patients often develop psychiatric symptoms. Anxiety, depression, and delirium frequently complicate the course of advancing illness (Breitbart 1987). In the following discussion, we focus on the unique aspects of psychiatric diagnosis and management of these symptoms in terminally ill cancer patients and highlight controversial areas such as suicide and euthanasia.

Anxiety

In this section, we focus on the unique aspects of control of anxiety—a common psychiatric symptom in terminally ill patients. (For a general discussion of the diagnosis and treatment of anxiety in cancer patients, see Chapter 1.) Terminally ill patients present with a complex mixture of physical and psychological symptoms in a context of a frightening reality. Thus the recognition of anxious symptoms requiring treatment can be challenging. Patients with anxiety complain of tension or restlessness, or they exhibit jitteriness, autonomic hyperactivity, vigilance, insomnia, distractibility, shortness of breath, numbness, apprehension, worry, or rumination. Often the physical or somatic manifestations of anxiety overshadow the psychological or cognitive ones and are the symptoms that patients most often present with (Holland 1989). The consultant must use these symptoms as a cue to enquire about the patients' psychological state, which is commonly one of fear, worry, or apprehension. The assumption that a high level of anxiety is inevitably encountered during the terminal phase of illness is neither helpful nor accurate for diagnostic and treatment purposes. In deciding whether to treat anxiety during the terminal phase of illness, the patients' subjective level of distress is the primary impetus for the initiation of treatment. Other considerations include problematic patient behavior such as noncompliance due to anxiety, family and staff reactions to patients' distress, and the balancing of the risks and benefits of treatment (Massie 1989).

Anxiety, like fever, is a symptom in this population that can have many etiologies. Anxiety may be encountered as a component of an adjustment disorder, panic disorder, generalized anxiety disorder, phobia, or agitated depression. However, in terminally ill cancer patients, symptoms of anxiety are most likely to arise from some medical complication of the illness or treatment such as organic anxiety disorder, delirium, or other organic mental disorders (Holland 1989; Massie 1989; Massie and Holland 1987). Hypoxia, sepsis, poorly controlled pain, and adverse drug reactions such as delirium, akathisia, or withdrawal states are specific entities that often present as anxiety. Patients who had been managed for long periods of time with relatively high doses of benzodiazepines or opioid analgesics for the control of anxiety or pain, often become tolerant or physically dependent on these drugs. During terminal phases of illness, when patients become less alert, there is a tendency to minimize the use of sedating medications. It is important to consider the need to slowly taper benzodiazepines and opioid analgesics to prevent acute withdrawal states. Withdrawal states in terminally ill patients often present first as agitation or anxiety and become clinically evident days later than might be expected in younger, healthier patients due to impaired metabolism. In dying patients, anxiety can represent impending cardiac or respiratory arrest, pulmonary embolism, electrolyte imbalance, or dehydration (Strain et al. 1981).

Despite the fact that anxiety in terminal illness commonly results from medical complications, it is important not to forget that psychological factors related to death and dying or existential issues play a role in anxiety, particularly in patients who are alert and not confused (Holland 1989). Patients frequently fear the isolation and separation of death. Claustrophobic patients may be afraid of the idea of being confined and buried in a coffin. These issues can be disconcerting to consultants who may find themselves at a loss for words that are consoling to such patients. Nonetheless, the clinician should not avoid eliciting these concerns, listening empathetically to them, and enlisting pastoral involvement when appropriate.

The specific treatment of anxiety in terminally ill patients often depends on etiology, presentation, and setting. An example of how the specific etiology of the anxious symptom is important is the case of hypoxia. Anxiety associated with hypoxia and dyspnea in a patient with diffuse lung metastases is most responsive to treatment with oxygen and opioid analgesics. If the same patient's presentation included hallucinations and agitation, a neuroleptic would be added to the regimen. In terms of setting, in the hospital an arterial blood gas could confirm the diagnosis and specific treatments would be administered. At home, on the other hand, such invasive diagnostics would likely be avoided or unavailable, and anxiety would be treated in nonspecific fashion using benzodiazepines.

The pharmacotherapy of anxiety in terminal illness involves the judicious use of the following classes of medications: benzodiazepines, neuroleptics, antihistamines, antidepressants, and opioid analgesics (Holland 1989; Massie 1989; Massie and Holland 1987). Benzodiazepines are the mainstays of the treatment of anxiety in terminally ill cancer patients. The shorter-acting benzodiazepines, such as lorazepam, oxazepam, and alprazolam, are safest in this population. Lorazepam and oxazepam are metabolized by conjugation in the liver and are most desirable for use in patients with hepatic disease. Alprazolam is metabolized through oxidative pathways in the liver and should be used with more caution in patients with hepatic damage. The selection of these shorter-acting drugs avoids toxic accumulation due to impaired metabolism in debilitated individuals (Hollister 1986).

The disadvantage of using short-acting benzodiazepines is that patients often experience breakthrough anxiety or end-of-dose failure. Such patients benefit from switching to longer-acting benzodiazepines such as diazepam or clonazepam. Dying patients often benefit from parenteral administration of these drugs. Common dosage regimens include lorazepam 0.5–2.0 mg po or iv every 3–6 hours, alprazolam 0.25–1.0 mg po three to four times a day, diazepam 2.5–10 mg po or iv every 3–6 hours, and clonazepam 1–2 mg po two to three times a day. Recently we have administered diazepam rectally in a saline solution to a dying patient who had no other route available and used dosages equivalent to oral regimens. Fears of causing respiratory depression should not prevent the clinician from using adequate dosages of benzodiazepines to control anxiety. The likelihood of respiratory depression is minimized when one uses shorter-acting drugs, increases the dosages in small increments, and ultimately switches to the longer-acting drugs.

Neuroleptics, such as thioridazine and haloperidol, are useful in the treatment of anxiety when benzodiazepines are not sufficient for symptom control (Massie 1989). They are also indicated when an organic etiology is suspected or when psychotic symptoms such as delusions or hallucinations accompany the anxiety. Typically, haloperidol 0.5–5 mg po or iv every 2–12 hours is sufficient to control anxious symptoms and avoid excessive sedation. Low-potency neuroleptics such as thioridazine (10–25 mg po tid) are effective anxiolytics and can help with insomnia and agitation. Neuroleptics are perhaps the safest class of anxiolytics in patients for whom there is legitimate concern regarding respiratory depression or compromise. Methotrimeprazine (10–20 mg im or iv qid) is a phenothiazine with unique analgesic and anxiolytic properties that is often used for the treatment of pain and anxiety in dying patients (Beaver et al. 1966). Its side effects include sedation, anticholinergic symptoms, and hypotension. Intravenous administration by slow infusion is preferable to avoid problems with hypotension. Chlorpromazine (12.5–50 mg po, im, or iv every 4–12 hours) has similar side effects that limit its application in this setting. However, it can be useful in patients for whom sedation is desirable.

With neuroleptics in general, it is important to be aware of extrapyramidal side effects (particularly when patients are taking additional neuroleptics for antiemetic purposes) and the remote possibility of neuroleptic malignant syndrome. Tardive dyskinesia is rarely a concern given the generally short-term usage and low dosages of these medications in this population (Breitbart 1986). Hydroxyzine is an antihistamine with mild anxiolytic, sedative, and analgesic properties. It is particularly useful when treating anxious, terminally ill cancer patients with pain. Hydroxyzine 100 mg given parenterally has analgesic potency equivalent to morphine 8 mg and potentiates the analgesic effects of morphine (Beaver and Feise 1976). **NOTE: Benzodiazepines may actually lower the pain threshold and probably should be used selectively in patients for whom pain is the primary problem.**

Tricyclic and heterocyclic antidepressants are the most effective treatment of anxiety accompanying depression and are helpful in treating panic disorder (Liebowitz 1985; Massie 1989); guidelines for their use are discussed in the section on depression below. Their usefulness is often limited in dying patients due to anticholinergic and sedative side effects. Very often the consultant is faced with the task of relieving symptoms in a short period of time, and therefore drugs that require 5–10 days to achieve therapeutic effect are unsatisfactory. For this reason, the use of buspirone as an anxiolytic is also limited in this population.

Opioid drugs such as the narcotic analgesics are primarily indicated for the control of pain. However, these drugs are also effective in the relief of dyspnea caused by cardiopulmonary processes and the anxiety associated with them. Opioid drugs are particularly useful in the treatment of dying patients who are in respiratory distress. Continuous intravenous infusions of morphine or other narcotic analgesics allow for careful titration and control of respiratory distress, anxiety, pain, and agitation (Portenoy et al. 1986). Often one must maintain the patient in a state of unresponsiveness to maximize comfort. When respiratory distress is not a major problem, it is preferable to use the opioid drugs solely for analgesic purposes and to add more specific anxiolytics (e.g., the benzodiazepines) to control concomitant anxiety. The following case example illustrates the importance of assessment in the management of anxiety in advanced disease:

Case 1

Mr. Q, a 54-year-old man with metastatic pancreatic cancer, was admitted to the hospital with severe nausea, vomiting, and dehydration.

His initial treatment included rehydration and a regimen of antiemetic therapy (metoclopramide 10 mg iv qid). On his second hospital day, he became agitated, diaphoretic, and dyspneic and complained of intense fear and anxiety. Diagnostic assessment revealed hypoxia secondary to pulmonary embolism. He was treated with a combination of nasal oxygen, thioridazine (25 mg po tid), and anticoagulant therapy resulting in prompt relief of the anxious symptoms. Four days later, he began to complain of restlessness, jitteriness, and intense anxiety. A reassessment revealed mild extrapyramidal symptoms including tremor and cogwheel rigidity. In addition, Mr. Q described an inner sense of restlessness that he could not relate to his current psychological state. A diagnosis of akathisia secondary to the combination of two dopamine-blocking neuroleptics (metoclopramide and thioridazine) was made. This was treated with lorazepam 1.0 mg iv tid and the lowering of the dosages of the neuroleptics, resulting in relief of all target symptoms.

Delirium

Delirium is common in patients with far-advanced cancer. Massie et al. (1983) found delirium in more than 75% of 20 terminally ill cancer patients they studied. (For a review of the management of delirium in cancer patients, see Chapter 2.) A standard approach for managing delirium in cancer patients includes a search for the underlying causes, correction of those factors, and management of the symptoms of delirium.

The treatment of delirium in dying cancer patients is unique however because 1) most often, the etiology of terminal delirium is multifactorial; 2) when a distinct cause is found, it is usually irreversible (e.g., hepatic failure or brain metastases); 3) workup may be limited by the setting (e.g, home and hospice); and 4) the consultant's focus is usually on the patients' comfort, and ordinarily helpful diagnostic procedures that are unpleasant or painful (e.g., computed tomography [CT] scan and lumbar puncture) may be avoided. When confronted with a delirium in terminally ill or dying cancer patients, a differential diagnosis should always be formulated (Adams et al. 1986); however, studies should be pursued only when a suspected factor can be identified easily and treated effectively. Irreversible etiologies that have no specific management should not be pursued. The following case example illustrates this approach:

Case 2

Mr. R, a 67-year-old man with widely metastatic end-stage multiple myeloma, was being cared for in a palliative care hospital. He had several pain syndromes secondary to metastatic bone disease that were well controlled on a stable regimen of opioid analgesics. He became incoherent, lethargic, and developed both visual and tactile hallucinations to which he was responding with facial contortions of fear. His medical history revealed two previous episodes of delirium. Each episode had been associated with hypercalcemia that had responded to both standard medical treatment to normalize the elevated serum calcium and haloperidol. Management here consisted of 1) a 24-hour companion to ensure safety and provide reassurance, 2) education and support of family, 3) laboratory studies that revealed a serum calcium of 13.4 mg/dl (normal 9.5 to 11.5 mg/dl), 4) haloperidol started at 1.0 mg given intravenously every 6 hours, and 5) hydration and diuresis with furosemide (Lasix). Over the ensuing 4 days, Mr. R became lucid and articulate, and serial laboratory studies documented a gradual normalization of the calcium. He died 7 weeks later of pneumonia.

In Case 2, the diagnostic workup was relatively painless, noninvasive, and targeted at a potentially reversible cause of delirium. Management of delirium in this case consisted of hydration, diuresis, and simultaneously administered neuroleptic. The treatment of delirium with neuroleptic medication often hastens recovery and relieves symptoms such as agitation, paranoia, hallucinations, and disorganized thinking.

The use of neuroleptics in the management of delirium in dying patients remains controversial in some circles. Some have argued that pharmacological interventions with neuroleptics or benzodiazepines are inappropriate in dying patients. Delirium is viewed as a natural part of the dying process that should not be altered. Another rationale often raised is that these patients are so close to death that aggressive treatment is unnecessary. Parenteral neuroleptics or sedatives may be mistakenly avoided because of exaggerated fears that they might hasten death through hypotension or respiratory depression. Many are unnecessarily pessimistic about the possible results of neuroleptic treatment for delirium. They argue that because the underlying pathophysiological process (e.g, hepatic or renal failure) often continues unabated, no improvement can be expected in the patients' mental status. There is also concern that neuroleptics or sedatives may worsen a delirium by making the patient more confused or sedated.

Clinical experience in managing delirium in dying cancer patients suggests that the use of neuroleptics in the management of agitation, paranoia, hallucinations, and altered sensorium is safe, effective, and quite appropriate (Adams et al. 1986; Massie and Holland 1987; Massie et al. 1983). Management of delirium on a case-by-case basis seems wisest. Agitated, delirious dying patients should probably be given neuroleptics to help restore calm. A "wait-and-see" approach, before using neuroleptics, may be most appropriate with patients who have a lethargic or somnolent presentation of delirium (Murray 1987). The consultant must educate staff and patients and weigh each of these issues in making the decision of whether to use pharmacological interventions for dying patients who present with delirium.

Haloperidol in low doses (1–3 mg) is usually effective in targeting agitation, paranoia, and fear. If an intravenous line is available, we prefer this route, as it facilitates rapid onset of medication effects. If intravenous access is unavailable, we suggest starting with intramuscular injections and switching to the oral route once the delirium is controlled. Clearly, in certain instances, pharmacological intervention is inappropriate, as the following example demonstrates:

Case 3

Ms. S, a 58-year-old elementary school teacher, was evaluated in the intensive care unit for visual hallucinations. She had refractory leukemia and was bleeding secondary to thrombocytopenia. Her husband of 35 years had died unexpectedly 6 weeks earlier. During the psychiatric consultation, she described episodic visual hallucinations in which she saw her dead husband lying next to her. She explained that these hallucinations were comforting as she felt less isolated when she "saw" her husband. The psychiatrist recommended no medication. Ms. S died without any agitation or fear 24 hours later.

As the following case example illustrates, the treatment of terminal delirium always includes the patient's family:

Case 4

The family of Ms. T, a 58-year-old woman with advanced, metastatic breast cancer, requested a psychiatric consultation because Ms. T was "not herself." She had been hospitalized because of poorly controlled pain secondary to multiple bone metastases. Large doses of intravenous hydromorphone (8 mg iv every 4 hours) were required for pain relief. Several other narcotic analgesics were intolerable because of their side effects. On this current analgesic regimen, she developed a lethargic delirium manifested by social withdrawal, incoherent babbling speech, reversal of sleep-wake cycle, and disorientation. The family maintained a constant vigil at her bedside as they felt her death was near. The family was particularly distressed by her profound withdrawal. She had been an outgoing woman who had coped extremely well with her illness and its treatment. Both family and medical staff were reluctant to make any changes in her pain medication as she had been in severe pain for several days before the current regimen had finally provided some relief. The consulting psychiatrist diagnosed a delirium, most likely due to the psychotomimetic effects of the opioid analgesic. Haloperidol 2 mg iv every 8 hours was prescribed. Within 24 hours Ms. T was oriented, coherent, and conversational. She was able once again to recognize her husband and daughters and to interact with them. Lethargy remained but did not worsen. Her family was able to converse with her over the next 10 days until her death.

In Case 4, haloperidol successfully treated the patient's disorganized thinking, regulated her sleep-wake cycle, and helped reorient her, partially clearing her sensorium. This intervention also allowed the patient to tolerate her current opioid analgesic regimen despite its psychotomimetic effects. More importantly, the patient became coherent and alert enough to communicate meaningfully with her family in her last days of life.

Depression

Depressed mood and sadness can be appropriate responses as terminally ill patients face death. These emotions can be manifestations of anticipatory grief over the impending loss of life, health, loved ones, and autonomy. The diagnosis of a major depressive syndrome in terminally ill patients often relies more on the psychological or cognitive symptoms of major depression (i.e., worthlessness, hopelessness, excessive guilt, and suicidal ideation), rather than on the neurovegetative or somatic signs and symptoms of major depression (Endicott 1984; Massie and Holland 1984; Plumb and Holland 1977). The presence of neurovegetative signs and symptoms of depression, such as fatigue, loss of energy, and other somatic symptoms, is often not helpful in establishing a diagnosis of depression in terminally ill patients. Terminal illness itself can produce many of these physical symptoms so characteristic of major depression in the physically healthy.

The strategy of relying on the psychological or cognitive signs and symptoms of depression for diagnostic specificity is itself not without pitfalls. How is the clinician to interpret feelings of hopelessness in dying patients when there is no hope for cure or recovery? Typically our practice is to explore feelings of hopelessness, worthlessness, or suicidal ideation in some detail. Although they lose hope of a cure, many dying patients are able to maintain hope that pain can be controlled. Hopelessness that is pervasive and accompanied by a sense of despair or despondency is more likely to represent a symptom of a depressive disorder (Massie and Holland 1984). Similarly, patients often state that they feel they are burdening their families unfairly, causing them great pain and inconvenience. Such beliefs are less likely to represent a symptom of depression than are patients' feelings that their lives have never had any worth or that they are being punished for evil things they have done. Suicidal ideation, even rather mild and passive forms, is very likely associated with significant degrees of depression in terminally ill cancer patients (Breitbart et al. 1987).

Supportive psychotherapy and pharmacotherapy are useful treatment approaches to depression in the terminally ill patient. Psychotherapy with a dying patient consists of active listening with supportive verbal interventions and the occasional interpretation (Cassem 1987). Despite the seriousness of the patient's plight, it is not necessary for the psychiatrist or psychologist to appear overly solemn or emotionally restrained. Often it is only the psychotherapist, of all the patient's caregivers, who is comfortable enough to converse lightheartedly and allow the patient to talk about his or her life and experiences, rather than focus solely on impending death. The dying patient who wishes to talk or ask questions about death should be allowed to do so freely, with the therapist maintaining an interested, interactive stance. It is not uncommon for the dying patient to benefit from pastoral counseling. If a chaplaincy service is available, it should be offered to the patient and family.

Tricyclic antidepressants and psychostimulants both have roles in the pharmacological treatment of depressed terminally ill patients (Massie and Holland 1984). Factors such as prognosis and the time frame for treatment may play important roles in determining the type of pharmacotherapy for depression. A depressed patient with several months of life expectancy can afford to wait the 10–14 days it may take to respond to a tricyclic antidepressant. The depressed dying patient with less than 3 weeks to live may do best with a rapid-acting psychostimulant. Patients who are within hours to days of death and in distress are likely to benefit most from the use of sedatives or narcotic analgesic infusions. Starting doses of the tricyclics are low, 10–25 mg, with dosages increased to between 25 mg and 75 mg.

Prescribing tricyclics (e.g., desipramine, nortriptyline, amitriptyline, and imipramine) based on plasma drug levels is often useful because medically ill patients in general, and those with far-advanced cancer in particular, are often found to have therapeutic plasma levels at modest dosages (Stoudemire and Fogel 1987). Moreover, typical regimens of the tricyclics (100–250 mg/day) can cause toxic effects in these patients, and plasma levels obtained on a serial basis can guide the physician in effective and safe administration. The side effects of the tricyclics are often troubling and occasionally serious. Plasma-level monitoring can ensure adequate treatment while minimizing the risk of side effects or toxicity (Preskorn and Jerkovich 1990). For patients who cannot take medications orally, most tricyclics are available as rectal suppositories, and some, such as amitriptyline, can be given as an intramuscular injection. Outside of the United States, certain tricyclics are given as intravenous infusion (Massie and Holland 1984).

Two newer antidepressants, fluoxetine and bupropion, deserve comment. Neither of these medications has been systematically studied in medically ill patients to date. Fluoxetine and its active metabolite, norfluoxetine, have long half-lives. The half-life of the parent compound averages 1–4 days and the metabolite 7–14 days. Also, since it has entered the market, there have been several reports of significant drug-drug interactions (Ciraulo and Shader 1990; Pearson 1990). Until it has been further studied in medically ill patients, we suggest cautious use of fluoxetine, particularly in debilitated patients for whom the long half-life may be more problematic. Bupropion may have a role in the treatment of psychomotor-retarded, depressed terminally ill patients because it has energizing effects similar to those of the stimulant drugs (Shopsin 1983). However, because of the increased incidence of seizures in patients with central nervous system disorders, bupropion has a limited role in the oncology population.

The psychostimulants offer an alternative pharmacological approach to the treatment of depression in terminally ill patients (Fernandez et al. 1987; Satel and Nelson 1989; Woods et al. 1986). These drugs have a more rapid onset of action than do the tricyclics and are often energizing. Thus they are particularly useful for patients who cannot tolerate the lethargy and weakness that frequently accompany advancing disease. Methylphenidate and amphetamine are given once a day in doses starting at 2.5–5.0 mg and increased as indicated. Many terminally ill patients respond to a single daily dose of 2.5 mg. A paranoid psychosis can occur as a side effect of stimulants, most often within 3 days of starting treatment. For patients who cannot swallow or digest pills, pemoline (a less widely used psychostimulant that comes in a chewable tablet form) can be chewed and absorbed through the buccal mucosa. The starting dose is usually 18.75 mg in the morning. Pemoline should be used with caution in patients with significant hepatic or renal impairment.

Suicide and Terminally Ill Patients

Cancer patients are at increased risk of suicide relative to the general population, particularly during the terminal stage of illness. Factors associated with increased risk of suicide in cancer patients are listed in Table 8–1 (Breitbart 1987). Patients with advanced illness are at high-

Table 8–1.   Cancer suicide vulnerability factors

Advanced illness and poor prognosis

Uncontrolled pain

Depression and hopelessness

Delirium and disinhibition

Loss of control and helplessness

Preexisting psychopathology

Prior suicide history and family history of suicide

Exhaustion and fatigue

Source.   Adapted from Breitbart W: "Cancer Pain and Suicide," in *Advances in Pain Research and Therapy,* Vol. 16. Edited by Foley KM, Bonica JJ, Ventafridda V. New York, Raven, 1990, p. 405. Used with permission.

est risk, perhaps because they are most likely to have cancer complications such as pain, depression, delirium, and deficit symptoms. Psychiatric disorders are frequently present in hospitalized cancer patients who are suicidal. A recent review (Breitbart 1987) of our psychiatric consultation data at Memorial Sloan-Kettering Cancer Center showed that 33% of suicidal cancer patients had a major depression, about 20% had a delirium, and 50% were diagnosed as having an adjustment disorder with both anxious and depressed features at the time of evaluation.

Cancer patients commit suicide most frequently in the advanced stages of disease (Bolund 1985a, 1985b; Farberow et al. 1963; Fox et al. 1982; Louhivuori and Hakama 1979). Of several hundred suicides studied by Farberow et al. (1963), 86% occurred in the preterminal or terminal stages of illness, despite greatly reduced physical capacity. Poor prognosis and advanced illness usually go hand-in-hand, so it is not surprising that in Sweden, patients who were expected to die within a matter of months were the most likely to commit suicide (Bolund 1985a, 1985b). Of 88 cancer patients who committed suicide, 14 had an uncertain prognosis, and 45 had a poor prognosis. With advancing disease, the incidence of significant cancer pain increases. Uncontrolled pain in cancer patients is a dramatically important risk factor for suicide. In several studies (Bolund 1985a, 1985b; Farberow et al. 1971), the vast majority of cancer patients who committed suicide had severe pain that was often inadequately controlled and poorly tolerated. The following case example illustrates the role of uncontrolled pain in suicide:

Case 5

Mr. U, a 56-year-old immigrant chef from Taiwan who spoke no English, was working in a Chinese-American restaurant when he developed oat-cell carcinoma of the lung. His illness had been unresponsive to therapy for over 6 months. His children accompanied him to the clinic one day, explaining that their father had taken an overdose of pills the night before. He had written a suicide note asking that his family forgive him and understand that he could not take the pain anymore. He had been disappointed when his attempt failed. When the psychiatrist evaluating the suicide attempt asked for more information about his pain, he said that he had been having extreme pain on the left side, especially in his ribs. No one, not his daughter, son-in-law (who interpreted), or his oncologist, was aware that he was in pain. He was receiving no analgesics. A chest X ray revealed metastases to several ribs. When Mr. U was informed that there were medications available that could diminish the pain and that the treatment team would vigorously attempt to control his pain, he was no longer suicidal. The difficulty in communication, combined with his stoic nature, had led him to feel that there was no other way out of a controllable pain problem except death.

Depression is a factor in 50% of all suicides; those suffering from depression are at 25 times greater risk of suicide than the general population (Guze and Robins 1970). The role depression plays in cancer suicide is equally significant. Approximately 25% of all cancer patients experience severe depressive symptoms, with about 6% fulfilling DSM-III criteria (American Psychiatric Association 1980) for the diagnosis of major depression (Bukberg et al. 1984; Derogatis et al. 1983; Plumb and Holland 1977). Among cancer patients with advanced illness and progressively impaired physical function, symptoms of severe depression rise to 77% (Bukberg et al. 1984).

Hopelessness is the key variable that links depression and suicide in the general population. Further, hopelessness is a significantly better predictor of completed suicide than is depression alone (Beck et al. 1975; Kovacs et al. 1975). With the typical cancer suicide being characterized by advanced illness and poor prognosis, hopelessness is commonly experienced. In Scandinavia, the highest incidence of suicide was found among cancer patients who were offered no further treatment and no further contact with the health care system (Bolund 1985a, 1985b; Louhivuori and Hakama 1979). Being left to face illness alone creates a sense of isolation and abandonment that is critical to the development of hopelessness.

The prevalence of organic mental disorders among cancer patients requiring psychiatric consultation has been found to range from 25% to 40% (Levine et al. 1978; Massie et al. 1979) and to be as high as 85% during the terminal stages of illness (Massie et al. 1983). Although earlier work (Farberow et al. 1963) suggested that delirium was a protective factor in regard to cancer suicide, our clinical experience has found these confusional states to be a major contributing factor in impulsive suicide attempts, especially in the hospital setting.

Loss of control and a sense of helplessness in the face of cancer are important factors in suicide vulnerability. Control refers to both the helplessness induced by symptoms or deficits caused by cancer or its treatments and the excessive need on the part of some patients to be in control of all aspects of living or dying. Farberow et al. (1963) noted that cancer patients who were accepting and adaptable were much less likely to commit suicide than were cancer patients who exhibited a need to be in control of even the most minute details of their care. This controlling trait may be prominent in some patients and cause distress with little provocation. However, it is not uncommon for cancer-related events to induce a great sense of helplessness even in patients who are not typically controlling individuals. Impairments or deficits induced by cancer or cancer treatments include loss of mobility, paraplegia, loss of bowel and bladder function, amputation, aphonia, sensory loss, and inability to eat or swallow. Most distressing to patients is the sense that they are losing control of their minds, especially when they are confused or sedated by medications. The risk of suicide is increased in cancer patients with such physical impairments, especially when accompanied by psychological distress and disturbed interpersonal relationships due to these deficit factors (Farberow et al. 1971).

Fatigue, in the form of exhaustion of physical, emotional, spiritual, financial, familial, communal, and other resources increases risk of suicide in cancer patients (Breitbart 1987). Cancer is now often a chronic illness. Increased survival is accompanied by increased numbers of hospitalizations, complications, and expense. Symptom control thus becomes a prolonged process with frequent advances and setbacks. The dying process also can become extremely long and arduous for all concerned. It is not uncommon for both family members and health care providers to withdraw prematurely from a cancer patient under these circumstances. A suicidal patient can thus feel even more isolated and abandoned. The presence of a strong support system for the patient that may act as an external control of suicidal behavior reduces risk of suicide among cancer patients significantly.

Holland (1982) has advised that it is extremely rare for a cancer patient to commit suicide without some degree of premorbid psychopathology that places him or her at increased risk. Farberow et al. (1963) described a large group of cancer patients who committed suicide as the "dependent dissatisfied." These patients were immature, demanding, complaining, irritable, hostile, and difficult ward management problems. Staff often felt manipulated by these patients and became irritable due to what they saw as excessive demands for attention. Suicide attempts or threats were often seen as "hysterical" or manipulative. Our consultation data on suicidal cancer patients showed that half had a diagnosable personality disorder (Breitbart 1987).

The frequency of suicide attempts among cancer patients has not been well studied. Although the frequency of suicidal thinking in the cancer setting may be in question, its relationship to suicide attempts or completions is clearer. Bolund (1985a, 1985b) reported that fully half of all Swedish cancer patients who committed suicide had previously conveyed suicidal thoughts or plans to their relatives. In addition, many of the completed suicides had been preceded by an attempted suicide. This is consistent with the statistics of suicide in general, which show that a previous suicide attempt greatly increases the risk of completed suicide (Dubovsky 1978; Murphy 1977). A family history of suicide is of increasing relevance in assessing suicide risk.

Frequency of Suicidal Ideation

Thoughts of suicide probably occur quite frequently, particularly in the setting of advanced cancer, and seem to act as a steam valve for feelings often expressed by patients: "If it gets too bad, I always have a way out." It has been our experience working with cancer patients that once a trusting and safe relationship develops, patients almost universally reveal that they have had occasionally persistent thoughts of suicide as a means of escaping the threat of being overwhelmed by cancer. Recent reports, however, suggest that suicidal ideation is relatively infrequent in cancer and is limited to patients who are significantly depressed. Silberfarb et al. (1980) found that only three of 146 breast cancer patients had suicidal thoughts, whereas none of the 100 cancer patients interviewed in a Finnish study expressed suicidal thoughts (Achte and Vanhkouen 1971). In a study conducted at St. Boniface Hospice in Winnipeg, Canada, Brown et al. (1986) found that only 10 of 44 terminally ill cancer patients were suicidal or desired an early death, and all 10 were suffering from clinical depression. At Memorial Sloan-Kettering Cancer Center, suicide risk evaluation accounted for 8.6% of psychiatric consultations, usually requested by staff in response to a patient verbalizing suicidal wishes (Breitbart 1987). We recently studied 185 cancer patients with pain at Memorial Sloan-Kettering Cancer Center and found that suicidal ideation occurred in 17% of the study population (see Saltzburg et al. 1989). The discrepancy between clinical impression and research conclusions may be due to the limitations of the research interview in eliciting reports of suicidal thinking.

Rational Suicide (Euthanasia)

In a survey (Helig 1988) of California physicians, 57% of those responding reported that they had been asked by terminally ill patients to hasten death. Persistent pain and terminal illness were the primary reasons for requesting physician-assisted euthanasia. What is the appropriate response to such a request?

The clinician in the oncology setting faces a dilemma when confronting the issue of suicide or euthanasia in the cancer patient. From the medical perspective, professional training reinforces the view of suicide as a manifestation of psychiatric disturbance to be prevented at all costs. However, from the philosophical perspective, many in our society view suicide in patients who face the distress of an often fatal and painful disease like cancer as "rational" and a means to regain control and maintain a "dignified death." An internal debate thus often takes place within the cancer care professional that is not dissimilar to the public debate that surrounds celebrated cases in which the rights of patients to terminate life-sustaining measures or receive active euthanasia are at issue.

The Humane and Dignified Death Act, a proposed law that would free doctors from criminal and civil liability if they participate in voluntary active euthanasia, did not appear on the 1988 California ballot because the sponsoring group (Americans Against Human Suffering) barely failed to get the required number of signatures. That group, an affiliate organization of the National Hemlock Society, did however undertake a survey (Helig 1988) of California physicians (as part of their efforts to build support for the act) that was quite revealing. Seventy percent of physicians who responded agreed that patients should have the option of active euthanasia in terminal illness. More than half of the physicians said that they would practice active voluntary euthanasia if it were legal. Twenty-three percent revealed that they already had practiced active euthanasia at least once in their careers. Of the 60% of physicians who indicated that they had been asked by patients with terminal illness to hasten death, nearly all agreed that such requests from patients can be described as "rational."

Public support for the "right to die" has been growing as well. Indeed, 65%–85% of the general population support a change in the law to permit physicians to help patients die, and there is greater acceptance by the public of suicide when pain and suffering coexist with terminal illness ("Quick and Painless Death" 1990).

Those of us who provide clinical care for cancer patients with pain and advanced illness are sympathetic to the goals of symptom control and relief of suffering, but are also obviously influenced by those who view suicide or active voluntary euthanasia as rational alternatives for patients already dying and in distress. Danger lies in the premature assumption that suicidal ideation or a request to hasten death in the cancer patient represents a "rational act" that is unencumbered by psychiatric disturbance. Accepted criteria for rational suicide (Siegel 1982; Siegel and Tuckel 1984) include the following: 1) the person must have clear mental processes that are unimpaired by psychological illness or severe emotional distress, such as depression; 2) the person must have a realistic assessment of the situation; and 3) the motives for the decision of suicide are understandable to most uninvolved observers. Clearly there are suicides that occur in the cancer setting that meet these criteria for rationality; however, a significant percentage, possibly the majority, do not by virtue of the fact that significant psychiatric comorbidity exists.

The patient who is knowledgeable about cancer and its treatment may opt to forego painful and invasive treatments that may prolong life for only a short period of time. Some observers, including at times medical staff and family members, might look on such a decision as a form of "passive suicide" (Breitbart 1987). However, the degree to which noncompliance or treatment refusal represents a deliberate decision to end life or constitutes "suicidal ideation" is unknown.

The President's Commission for the Study of Ethical Problems in Medicine and Biomedical and Behavioral Research (1983) concluded that competent and informed patients were entitled to make decisions about whether life-sustaining treatment might be undertaken or not. Thus a patient who is informed and competent can refuse a cancer treatment. Such a refusal does not necessarily represent "suicide" and should not be viewed as a psychiatric issue, per se; rather, it is a medical-ethical matter in which the mental health professional does have an important role to play.

In such circumstances, the psychiatrist or psychologist is often the professional most expert in assessing the competence of the individual refusing treatment. In addition, a decision on the part of a patient to refuse potentially helpful cancer treatment is often unpopular with medical staff and family. The oncologist, for example, has an investment in sustaining life and using his or her skills. He or she may regard the patient's decision to refuse treatment as premature if his or her emphasis is on prolongation of life as opposed to quality of life. Fortunately, oncologists today have a growing appreciation for the value of quality of life and are sensitive to the "rationality" of the patient's decision to forego treatment that has little chance of improving quality of life. Family members often have an investment in the patient's engaging in life-prolonging treatment at all costs. They may be reluctant to face the loss of their loved one and may oppose the patient's decision to forego treatment and prepare for death. It is therefore our role as psychiatrists and psychologists to intervene with staff and family and to act as an advocate for the patient. The oncologist can be helped to see that he or she has a valuable role in palliative care. The family members can be helped to confront and accept the inevitability of the impending loss.

By reviewing the current research data on cancer suicide and the role of factors such as pain, depression, and delirium, we hope to provide a factual framework on which to base guidelines for managing this vulnerable group of patients.

Management of Suicidal, Terminally Ill Cancer Patients

Assessment of suicide risk and appropriate intervention are critical. Early and comprehensive psychiatric involvement with high-risk individuals can often avert suicide in the cancer setting (Dubovsky 1978). A careful evaluation (Table 8–2) includes a search for the meaning of suicidal thoughts, as well as an exploration of the seriousness of the risk. The clinician's ability to establish rapport and elicit a patient's thoughts are essential as he or she assesses history, degree of intent, and quality of internal and external controls. The clinician must listen sympathetically, not appearing critical or stating that such thoughts are inappropriate. Allowing the patient to discuss suicidal thoughts often decreases the risk of suicide. The myth that asking about suicidal thoughts "puts the idea in their head," is one that should be dispelled, especially in the cancer setting (McKegney and Lange 1971). Patients often reconsider and reject the idea of suicide when the physician acknowledges the legitimacy of their option and the need to retain a sense of control over aspects of their death.

The cancer suicide vulnerability factors listed in Table 8–1 should be used as a guide to evaluation and management. Once the setting has been made secure, assessment of relevant mental status and adequacy of pain control can begin. Analgesics, neuroleptics, or antidepressant drugs should be used when appropriate to treat agitation, psychosis, major depression, or pain. Underlying causes of delirium or pain should be addressed specifically when possible. Initiation of a crisis-intervention–oriented psychotherapeutic approach, mobilizing as much of the patient's support system as possible, is important. A close family member or friend should be involved to support the patient, provide information, and assist in treatment planning. Psychiatric hospitalization can sometimes be helpful but is usually not desirable in terminally ill patients. Thus the medical hospital or home is the setting in which management most often takes place. Although it is appropriate to intervene when medical or psychiatric factors are clearly the driving

Table 8–2. Evaluation of suicidal cancer patients

Establish rapport with an empathic approach.

Obtain patient's understanding of illness and present symptoms.

Assess mental status (internal control).

Assess vulnerability variables (pain control).

Assess support system (external control).

Obtain history of prior emotional problems or psychiatric disorders.

Obtain family history.

Record prior suicide threats and attempts.

Assess suicidal thinking, intent, and plans.

Evaluate need for one-to-one nurse in hospital or companion at home.

Formulate treatment plan (immediate and long term).

Source. Adapted from Breitbart W: "Cancer Pain and Suicide," in *Advances in Pain Research and Therapy,* Vol. 16. Edited by Foley KM, Bonica JJ, Ventafridda V. New York, Raven, 1990, p. 409. Used with permission.

force in a cancer suicide, there are circumstances in which usurping control from the patient and family with overly aggressive intervention may be less helpful. This is most evident in patients with advanced illness where comfort and symptom control are the primary concerns.

The goal of the intervention should not be to prevent suicide at all costs, but to prevent suicide that is driven by desperation. Prolonged suffering caused by poorly controlled symptoms leads to such desperation, and it is the consultant's role to provide effective management of such problems as an alternative to suicide for cancer patients.

Controlling Physical Symptoms

Although the diagnosis and treatment of pain in patients with advanced cancer is of paramount importance, other troublesome physical symptoms (Table 8–3) must also be aggressively treated in efforts aimed at the enhancement of patients' quality of life (Bruera 1990). The deleterious influence of uncontrolled pain on a patient's psychological state is often intuitively understood and recognized; however, physical symptoms other than pain can go undetected and cause significant emotional distress. This distress often dissipates when effective management is instituted. In a recent study, Coyle et al. (1990) reported that 70% of terminally ill patients have three or more physical symptoms other than pain. This finding replicates those of earlier articles (e.g., Levy and Catalano 1985) that elucidated the multiple problems facing terminally ill patients. These symptoms must be assessed by the psy-

Table 8–3.   Physical symptoms in terminally ill cancer patients

Very common (40%–70%)	Less common (less than 10%)
Pain	Dysphagia
Constipation	Pulmonary congestion
Weakness	Dry and/or sore mouth
Anorexia	Decubitus
Weight Loss	
Common (10%–40%)	
Dyspnea	
Nausea and/or vomiting	
Insomnia	
Lethargy and/or sedation	

chologist or psychiatrist concerned with the assessment and treatment of affective and other syndromes in the terminally ill population. In the following sections, we discuss cancer pain and other physical symptoms and their management.

Cancer Pain

Pain is a common problem for cancer patients, with approximately 70% of patients experiencing severe pain at some point in the course of their illness (Foley 1985). Twycross and Lack (1983) have suggested that 25% of cancer patients die in severe pain. There is considerable variability in the prevalence of pain among different types of cancer. For example, approximately 5% of leukemia patients experience pain during the course of their illness as compared to 50%–75% of patients with tumors of the lung, gastrointestinal tract, or genitourinary system (Foley 1979). Patients with cancers of the bone or cervix have been found to have the highest prevalence of pain, with as many as 85% of patients experiencing significant pain during the course of their illness (Foley 1979). Yet, despite its prevalence, studies (Foley 1985; Marks and Sachar 1973) have shown that pain is frequently underdiagnosed and inadequately treated.

Pain is best conceptualized as a psychological experience involving nociception, pain perception, and pain behaviors. Thus the experience of pain is not limited to nociception alone. Psychological variables, such as the meaning of pain, fear of death, perception of control, and sense of hopelessness, can all greatly influence the individual's experience of cancer pain and of suffering in general (Breitbart 1989). For the cancer patient, pain is often distressing and demoralizing, greatly contributing to suffering.

Types of cancer pain.   There are three basic types of cancer pain described: somatic, visceral, and neuropathic (or deafferentation). The etiology, characteristics, underlying mechanisms, and management of each of these types of cancer pain can be quite distinct (Table 8–4). Somatic pain is thought to be mediated by the activation of nociceptors—receptors that are sensitive to tissue-damaging stimuli. Typically constant, aching or gnawing, and rather well localized, the pain associated with cancer that has metastasized to bone is an example of somatic pain. Visceral pain is also thought to be initiated by activation

Table 8–4. Characteristics, mechanisms, examples, and management of the three types of cancer pain

Type of pain	Characteristics	Mechanisms	Examples	Management
Somatic	Constant, aching, and gnawing; well localized	Activation of nociceptors	Metastases to bone	Treat tumor; narcotic analgesics; ± nerve blocks; ± cordotomy; ± NSAIDs
Visceral	Constant and aching; poorly localized; referred to cutaneous sites	Activation of nociceptors; ± autonomic component	Pancreatic cancer; liver or lung metastases with referred shoulder pain	Treat tumor; narcotic analgesics; ± cordotomy; ± sympathetic blocks; ± NSAIDS
Neuropathic	Shooting, shock-like paroxysms; burning; aching: dysesthesia	Nonnociceptive; paroxysmal discharges in the PNS and CNS; autonomic component	Brachial and lumbosacral plexopathies; postsurgical syndromes; phantom limb	Narcotic analgesics; tricyclic antidepressants; TENS; ± treat tumor

Note. NSAIDs = nonsteroidal anti-inflammatory drugs; PNS = peripheral nervous system; CNS = central nervous system; TENS = transcutaneous electrical nerve stimulation; ± = possibly relevant or indicated.

of nociceptors. Its characteristics are similar to somatic pain except that visceral pain tends to be more poorly localized and is frequently referred to cutaneous sites. Pain experienced with carcinoma of the pancreas or bowel obstruction are examples of visceral pain. Neuropathic or deafferentation pain occurs after nerve damage, either in the peripheral or central nervous systems. Such injury can result from tumor compression of nerve or spinal cord. Surgery, chemotherapeutic agents, or radiation therapy can also damage nerves or nerve plexuses causing neuropathic pain. Neuropathic pain is characterized by burning, aching, constricting, or paroxysms of shooting, shock-like, lancinating pain. These pains are often accompanied by dysesthesias and other evidence of altered nerve function caused by nerve damage.

Types of cancer pain patients. Foley (1985) described five types of patients with cancer pain: 1) patients with acute cancer-related pain, 2) patients with chronic cancer-related pain, 3) patients with preexisting chronic pain and cancer-related pain, 4) patients with preexisting substance abuse and cancer-related pain, and 5) dying patients with pain. Acute cancer-related pain, such as is seen with postoperative pain or pain caused by chemotherapy-induced stomatitis, is generally abrupt in onset, time-limited in duration, and often quite successfully managed with an adequate regimen of narcotic analgesics. Chronic cancer-related pain, defined as pain of 3–6 months in duration or longer, is often more difficult to treat effectively, especially as underlying disease progresses. Both acute and chronic cancer-related pain can result from direct tumor infiltration of soft tissue (bone and nerve) or from cancer therapy itself.

Patients with cancer-related pain who have preexisting chronic pain or substance abuse can be quite complicated to treat and can benefit from early psychiatric consultation. Patients with chronic pain, who then develop a cancer-related pain, bring along a longstanding set of difficulties that require active participation of psychiatry and psychology in their care. Such patients have a high incidence of depression, personality disorder, and occasionally substance abuse. The meaning of pain and the expression of pain, both verbally and through behaviors, are of particular significance when working with this group of patients. The treatment of patients with a prior history of substance abuse requires attention to important pharmacological and psychological factors. For example, patients who use opioids chronically (either illicitly or through methadone maintenance) are at risk for opioid withdrawal should the treatment team fail to prescribe an appropriate opioid regimen. Patients maintained on methadone are also at risk for undertreatment of cancer pain if their physiological tolerance to opioids is not taken into account. Our experience has helped us develop some practical recommendations:

1. Take physiological and pharmacological factors into account so that cancer pain can be managed adeptly.
2. Choose one physician to be responsible for pain assessment and therapy to minimize certain patients' manipulativeness.
3. Avoid the temptation to make major changes in the patient's substance abuse treatment (i.e., adding new agents or tapering old ones) during the stressful period of cancer therapy.

Even when these recommendations are followed, the treatment of the drug-abusing cancer pain patient poses a major challenge (Breitbart and Holland 1990; Macaluso et al. 1988).

The fifth and final type of patient with cancer-related pain is the patient in the terminal stages of illnesses who is dying. Treatment efforts for patients in this group should be directed primarily at providing comfort, while allowing them to function at a level acceptable to them and family members. The preferred balance of pain relief and level of alertness is a highly individual issue. For some patients, any experience of pain may signal the imminence of death and thus produces marked emotional distress. For such patients, pain relief is such a clear priority that they are willing to tolerate side effects such as sedation. For other patients, excessive sedation or confusion is experienced as so isolating and distressing that they prefer to tolerate some discomfort while maintaining valued contact with their loved ones.

Cancer pain syndromes.   Foley and colleagues (Elliot and Foley 1989; Foley 1979, 1987; Portenoy 1989) have also conceptualized cancer pain from the perspective of etiology. These cancer pain syndromes are outlined in Table 8–5. Most of these pain syndromes stem from direct tumor involvement. In a survey of patients with advanced cancer, Twycross and Lack (1983) found that 80% of patients experience more than one form of pain, and more than 33% experience four or more types of pain at any one time. As Foley (1987) pointed out, the cancer pain patient rarely has a single pain syndrome; rather, diagnosis and recognition of the totality of the range of cancer pain syndromes is essential for effective pain management.

Management of Cancer Pain

Assessment issues

The initial step in pain management is a comprehensive assessment of pain symptoms. A description of the qualitative features of the pain, its time course, and any maneuvers that increase or decrease pain intensity

Table 8–5.   Pain syndromes in patients with cancer

Pain syndromes associated with direct tumor infiltration (70%)
   Tumor infiltration of bone
   Tumor infiltration of soft tissue
   Tumor infiltration of nerve
      Brachial, lumbar, and sacral plexopathies
      Epidural spinal cord compression
Pain syndromes associated with cancer therapy (25%)
   Postsurgery syndromes
      Postmastectomy syndrome
      Postthoracotomy syndrome
      Phantom limb syndrome
   Chemotherapy-associated syndromes
      Peripheral neuropathy
      Postherpetic neuralgia
      Aseptic necrosis of femoral head
   Postradiation syndromes
      Radiation fibrosis of neural plexus (i.e., brachial)
      Radiation myelopathy
      Radiation-induced bone necrosis
Pain syndromes not associated with cancer (5%)
   Diabetic neuropathy
   Osteoarthritis and osteoporosis

---

should be obtained. In addition, detailed medical, neurological, and psychosocial assessments (including a history of substance use or abuse) must be completed. When possible, family members should be interviewed. During this assessment, cancer pain should be aggressively treated, and pain complaints and psychosocial issues should be subject to an ongoing process of reevaluation (Portenoy and Foley 1989).

The mental health professional working in the oncology setting must have a working knowledge of the etiology and treatment of cancer pain. This would include an understanding of the different types of cancer pain patients and syndromes discussed above, as well as a familiarity with the parameters of appropriate pharmacological treatment. Not uncommonly, the mental health professional is the first person to be informed of the pain complaint. The pain assessment in such instances may be complicated by comorbid psychiatric symptoms, such as depression or suicidal ideation. A close collaboration with the patient's oncologist or neurologist is essential to the successful treatment of cancer pain.

An important element in assessment of pain is the concept that assessment be continuous and repeated over the course of pain treatment. There are essentially three aspects of cancer pain that require ongoing evaluation: 1) pain intensity, 2) pain relief, and 3) mood state or psychological distress (Elliott and Foley 1990). The Memorial Pain Assessment Card (MPAC) (Fishman et al. 1987) is a helpful clinical tool that allows patients to report their pain experience. The MPAC consists of visual analog scales that measure pain intensity, pain relief, and mood. Patients can complete the MPAC in less than 30 seconds. Patients' report of pain intensity, pain relief, and present mood state provides the essential information required to help guide their pain management.

Pharmacological interventions

Foley and colleagues (Foley 1985; Foley and Inturrisi 1987; Inturrisi 1989; Portenoy 1990) have described the indications for and use of three classes of analgesic drugs in the cancer setting: 1) nonopioid analgesics (e.g., acetaminophen, aspirin, and other nonsteroidal anti-inflammatory drugs [NSAIDs]), 2) opioid analgesics (of which morphine is the standard), and 3) adjuvant analgesics (e.g., antidepressants and anticonvulsants). The World Health Organization's (WHO) Cancer Pain Relief Program (1986) has advocated an approach to the use of these analgesic drugs, which it has described as the three-step "analgesic ladder." Patients with mild cancer pain are managed with nonopioid analgesics such as the NSAIDs. Patients with moderate to severe pain move on to the second step on the analgesic ladder and should receive a weak opioid (e.g., codeine or oxycodone) in combination with a NSAID. Patients with severe pain who fail step two should go on to step three and receive a strong opioid analgesic (e.g., morphine) with or without a NSAID. Adjuvant analgesics may be used additionally at any one of the three steps of the analgesic ladder.

Nonopioid analgesics. The nonopioid analgesics are prescribed principally for mild to moderate pain or to augment the analgesic effects of narcotic analgesics in the treatment of severe pain. Characteristics of the nonopioid analgesics (as well as the weaker opioids) used for mild to moderate pain are described in Table 8–6. These drugs are especially useful in the treatment of patients who have pain from bone metastases (Brodie 1974; Bruera 1990). The analgesic effect of the NSAIDs appears to stem from their inhibition of cyclooxygenase and the subsequent reduction of prostaglandins in the tissues (Kantor 1984).

Opioid analgesics. Opioid analgesics are the mainstay of the pharmacological treatment of cancer patients with moderate to severe pain (Table 8–7). The following principles are useful in guiding the appropriate use of opioid analgesics for cancer pain (Foley and Inturrisi 1987; Inturrisi 1989; Portenoy 1990):

1. Choose an appropriate drug.
2. Start with the lowest dose possible.
3. Titrate the dose.
4. Use "as-needed" doses selectively.
5. Use an appropriate route of administration.
6. Be aware of equivalent analgesic doses.
7. Use a combination of drugs.
8. Be aware of tolerance.
9. Understand physical and psychological dependence.

Table 8–6.   Characteristics of oral analgesics for mild to moderate pain

Analgesic (by class)	Starting dose (mg)	Duration (hours)	Plasma half-life (hours)	Comments
Nonsteroidal				
Aspirin	650	4–6	4–6	The standard for comparison among nonopioid analgesics
Ibuprofen	400–600	—	—	Like aspirin, can inhibit platelet function
Choline magnesium trisalicylate	700–1500	8–12	—	Essentially no hematologic or gastrointestinal side effects
Weaker opioids				
Codeine	32–65	3–4	3–4	Metabolized to morphine, often used to suppress cough in patients at risk of pulmonary bleed
Oxycodone	5–10	3–4	—	Available as single agent and in combination with aspirin or acetaminophen
Propoxyphene	65–130	4–6	12	Toxic metabolite norpropoxyphene accumulates with repeated dosing

We have compiled a list of ten "clinical pearls" (Table 8–8) that are used in teaching the principles of cancer pain management to physicians and nurses at Memorial Sloan-Kettering Cancer Center.

In choosing the appropriate opioid analgesic for cancer pain, Portenoy (1990) highlighted six important considerations: 1) opioid class, 2) "weak" versus "strong" opioids, 3) pharmacokinetic characteristics, 4) duration of analgesic effect, 5) favorable prior response, and 6) opioid side effects.

Opioid analgesics are divided into two classes, the agonists and the agonist-antagonists, based on their affinity to opioid receptors. Morphine and most of the other opioid analgesics listed in Table 8–7 are agonist drugs. Pentazocine, butorphanol, and nalbuphine are examples of opioid analgesics with mixed agonist-antagonist properties. These drugs can reverse opioid effects and precipitate an opioid withdrawal syndrome in patients who are opioid tolerant or dependent. They are of limited use in the management of chronic cancer pain where the advantages of the agonist-antagonist opioids (a lower abuse or addiction potential) are less relevant. Buprenorphine, a partial agonist, may be appropriate for cancer pain (in its available sublingual form) for selected patients who are not opioid tolerant (Portenoy 1990). Oxycodone and codeine are the so-called weaker opioid analgesics and are thus not first-line agents for patients with severe, intractable pain. Oxycodone is often prescribed as a 5-mg oral dose with either aspirin or acetaminophen. More severe pain is best managed with morphine or another of the stronger opioid analgesics, such as hydromorphone, methadone, or levorphanol.

A basic understanding of the pharmacokinetics of the opioid analgesics is important for the mental health professional treating terminally ill cancer patients with pain (Inturrisi 1989). Opioid analgesics with long half-lives, such as methadone and levorphanol, require approximately 5 days to achieve a steady state. Despite their long half-lives, the duration of analgesia that they provide is considerably shorter (i.e., most patients will require administration of the drug every 4–6 hours). Because both methadone and levorphanol tend to accumulate with early initial dosing, delayed effects of toxicity can develop (primarily sedation and more rarely respiratory depression). Because of this unique profile, methadone is not recommended as first-line pain management, especially in elderly cancer patients.

The duration of analgesic effects of opioid analgesics varies con-

Table 8–7. Characteristics of narcotic analgesics for moderate to severe cancer pain

Analgesic	Route	Equianalgesic dose (mg)	Analgesic onset (hours)	Analgesic durations (hours)	Plasma half-life (hours)	Comments
Morphine (MS Contin)	po	60	1–1½	4–6	2–4	Standard of comparison for the narcotic analgesics. Now available in long-acting oral sustained-release preparations.
	im, iv, sc	10	½ –1	4–6	3–4	
Hydromorphone (Dilaudid)	po	7.5	½ –1	3–4	2–3	Short half-life may be preferable for elderly patients. Available in rectal suppository form and high-potency injectable forms.
	im, iv	1.5	¼ –½	3–4	2–3	
Methadone (Dolophine)	po	20	½ –1	4–6	15–30	Long half-life tends to accumulate and cause sedation with initial dosing, requiring careful titration. Good oral potency.
	im, iv	10	½ –1	—	15–30	

Levorphanol (Levo-Dromoran)	po	4	1–1½	4–6	12–16	Long half-life; requires careful dose titration in first week. Note that analgesic duration is considerably less than plasma half-life.
	im	2	½–1	4–5	12–16	
Meperidine (Demerol)	po	300	1–1½	4–6	3–4	Active toxic metabolite, normeperidine, tends to accumulate (plasma half-life of 12–16 hours), especially with renal impairment and in elderly patients, causing delirium, myoclonus, and seizures.
	im	75	½–1	4–5	3–4	
Buprenorphine (Buprenex)	sl	0.8	—	4–6	—	Partial agonist-antagonist, may precipitate opioid withdrawal in tolerant patients.
	im	0.4	—	4–6	—	

Note. po = oral; im = intramuscular; iv = intravenous; sl = sublingual; sc = subcutaneous.

siderably (Tables 8–6 and 8–7). Oxycodone will often provide only 3 hours of relief, and it must be prescribed on a 3-hour continuous basis (not as needed). Methadone and levorphanol may provide up to 6 hours of analgesia. There is individual variation in the metabolism of opioid

Table 8–8.   Cancer pain: ten clinical pearls

1. Administer analgesics on a fixed-time interval as well as an on-demand (rescue) basis.

2. Drug abuse is typically not a concern in the treatment of cancer pain in patients without history of substance abuse.

3. Be aware of equianalgesic doses when switching from one narcotic to another, or from one route to another.

4. The duration of analgesic effect is variable in each individual and is not always the same as the drug's serum half-life (e.g., methadone has 4–6 hours of analgesia, but its half-life is 12–32 hours).

5. There is no maximum dose of morphine (no ceiling effect for narcotic analgesia).

6. Meperidine (Demerol) is useful for post-op and other acute pain but is not advised for the treatment of chronic cancer pain. Accumulation of active toxic metabolite, normeperidine, produces central nervous system excitation and delirium. Contraindicated in patients with renal dysfunction.

7. If opioid side effects develop, consider changing to a different opioid drug.

8. Consider routes of drug administration other than the oral (i.e., intravenous, subcutaneous, epidural, and intrathecal) for increased efficacy or to minimize side effects.

9. Multimodal therapy is often useful. Combine pharmacotherapy with anesthetic, neurosurgical, rehabilitative, stimulatory (transcutaneous electrical nerve stimulation [TENS]), and psychological approaches.

10. Adjuvant analgesics (e.g., antidepressants and stimulants) can help potentiate narcotic analgesia and can improve mood, sleep, and oversedation.

analgesics, and there can be significant differences between individuals in drug absorption and disposition. These differences lead to a need for alterations in dosing, route of administration, and scheduling for maximum analgesia in individual patients. Although parenteral administration (i.e., intravenous, intramuscular, and subcutaneous) will yield a faster onset of pain relief, the duration of analgesia is shorter. For example, a patient started on intramuscular morphine might require administration every 3 hours. Once pain is under better control, for various reasons (e.g., discharge home) it may be desirable to have the patient switch to oral morphine. The patient might then require the drug every 4 hours. A longer-acting oral morphine preparation (MS Contin) is available that provides up to 8 hours of analgesia, minimizing the number of daily doses required for the control of cancer pain.

The adequate treatment of cancer pain also requires consideration of the equianalgesic doses of opioid drugs that are generally calculated using morphine as a standard (Table 8–7). Cross-tolerance is not complete among these drugs, therefore one-half to two-thirds of the equianalgesic dose of the new drug should be given as the starting dose when switching from one opioid to another (Foley and Inturrisi 1987). For example, if a patient receiving 20 mg of parenteral morphine is to be switched to hydromorphone, the equianalgesic dose of parenteral hydromorphone would be 3.0 mg. Thus the starting dose of parenteral hydromorphone should be approximately 1.5–2 mg. There is also considerable variability in the parenteral-to-oral ratios among the opioid analgesics. Both levorphanol and methadone have 1:2 intramuscular/oral ratios, whereas morphine has a 1:6 and hydromorphone a 1:5 intramuscular/oral ratio. Failure to appreciate these dosage differences in route of administration can lead to inadequate pain control.

Regular ("standing") scheduling of the opioid analgesics is the foundation of adequate pain control. It is preferable to prevent the return of pain as opposed to treating pain as it reoccurs. "As-needed" orders for chronic cancer pain often create a struggle between patient, family, and staff that is easily avoided by regular administration of opioid analgesics. The typical prescribing of methadone is a notable exception. It is often initially prescribed on an as-needed basis to determine the patient's total daily requirement and to minimize toxicity (due to its long half-life).

The concepts of opioid tolerance, physical dependence, and psychological dependence or drug abuse are often misunderstood. "Tolerance" is defined as the need for higher doses of opioid to maintain an effect. Tolerance to various opioid effects occurs at different rates, with tolerance to respiratory depression often occurring early. Escalation of opioid dose for analgesia in cancer pain is usually a function of developing tolerance or, more commonly, of the progression of underlying disease (Foley 1985). Physical dependence is related to opioid tolerance and is characterized by the development of an abstinence syndrome on abrupt withdrawal of the opioid or with administration of an opioid antagonist. Psychological dependence or drug abuse ("addiction") refers to a behavioral syndrome characterized by drug craving; concern with acquiring the drug, often from multiple physicians; and use for purposes other than pain control. Cancer pain patients without a prior history of drug abuse are at low risk for developing such problems when taking opioid analgesics for pain (Foley 1985; Macaluso et al. 1988). It is often helpful when the consultant educates nonpsychiatric physicians so that they can make these distinctions.

Although the opioids are extremely effective analgesics, their side effects are common and can be minimized if anticipated in advance (Inturrisi 1989). Sedation is a common central nervous system side effect, especially during the initiation of treatment. Sedation usually resolves after patients have been maintained on a steady dosage. Persistent sedation can be alleviated with a psychostimulant, such as dextroamphetamine, pemoline, or methylphenidate. All are prescribed in divided doses in early morning and at noon. Additionally, psychostimulants can improve depressed mood and enhance analgesia (Breitbart and Holland 1990; Bruera et al. 1987). Delirium, of either an agitated or a somnolent variety, can also occur in patients on opioid analgesics and is usually accompanied by attentional deficits, disorientation, and perceptual disturbances (e.g., visual hallucinations and, more commonly, illusions). Myoclonus and asterixis are often early signs of neurotoxicity that accompany the course of opioid-induced delirium. Meperidine (Demerol) when administered chronically, in patients with renal impairment, can lead to a delirium due to accumulation of the neuroexcitatory metabolite normeperidine (Kaiko et al. 1983).

Opioid-induced delirium can be alleviated through the implementation of three possible strategies: 1) lowering the dose of the opioid drug presently in use, 2) changing to a different opioid, or 3) treating the delirium with low doses of high-potency neuroleptics such as haloperidol. The third strategy is especially useful for agitation and clears the sensorium (Breitbart 1989). For agitated states, intravenous haloperidol in doses starting at 1–2 mg is useful, with rapid escalation of dose if no effect is noted. Gastrointestinal side effects of opioid analgesics are common. The most prevalent are nausea, vomiting, and constipation (Portenoy 1987). Concomitant therapy with prochlorperazine for nausea is sometimes effective. Because all opioid analgesics are not tolerated in the same manner, switching to another narcotic can be helpful if an antiemetic regimen fails to control nausea. Constipation caused by narcotic effects on gut receptors is a problem frequently encountered, and it tends to be responsive to the regular use of senna derivatives. A careful review of medications is imperative because anticholinergic drugs such as the tricyclic antidepressants can worsen opioid-induced constipation and cause bowel obstruction. Respiratory depression is a worrisome but rare side effect of the opioid analgesics. Respiratory difficulties can almost always be avoided if two general principles are adhered to: 1) start opioid analgesics in low doses in opioid-naive patients and 2) be cognizant of relative potencies when switching opioid analgesics, routes of administration, or both.

Adjuvants. Adjuvant analgesics are the third class of medications frequently prescribed for the treatment of cancer and noncancer pain. The most commonly used adjuvant analgesics in the treatment of cancer pain are the tricyclic antidepressants (Breitbart 1989; Breitbart and Holland 1990). The tricyclics have been empirically studied in patients with both chronic noncancer and cancer pain and have been used extensively in hospices (Walsh and Saunders 1984). The tricyclics are particularly valuable in the treatment of neuropathic pain syndromes such as diabetic neuropathy, postherpetic neuralgia, and phantom limb pain (pain experienced in an amputated limb). The analgesic action of the tricyclic antidepressants has been empirically demonstrated to be independent of their antidepressant effects (Spiegel et al. 1983). Although their precise mechanism of analgesic action is unknown, potentiates of the serotonergic system have been hypothesized to be central to their analgesic properties (Breitbart 1989). Tricyclic antidepressants increase the analgesic effects of opioid analgesics and so are quite useful in combination with narcotic analgesics in the management of cancer pain (Walsh 1986).

Amitriptyline is the most studied tricyclic antidepressant for the treatment of pain and is quite effective. Its utility can be limited due to anticholinergic side effects that can exacerbate the constipation, dry mouth, and other undesirable effects with which terminally ill cancer patients must often struggle. Nortriptyline can often be substituted for amitriptyline with fewer resultant side effects. Other frequently used adjuvant analgesics are agents from a variety of classes, including phenothiazines, psychostimulants, anticonvulsants, antihistamines, corticosteroids, and oral local anesthetics (Breitbart and Holland 1990; Bruera et al. 1989; Portenoy 1990).

Anorexia and Weight Loss

Cancer patients and their families find weight loss demoralizing, perplexing, and distressing. Weight loss and anorexia in terminally ill patients are complex problems that can arise from a number of sources. Among the chief sources of weight loss in the terminally ill population are decreased nutritional intake, hypercatabolic states, and malabsorption syndromes (Levy and Catalano 1985). The anorexia encountered in advanced illness is often due to specific physical difficulties; poorly controlled pain, mouth discomfort, dysphagia, nausea, and constipation are a few of the numerous factors frequently involved. Less frequent causes of anorexia include compression of the stomach (from hepatomegaly or ascites), hepatic failure, or metabolic abnormalities, such as hyponatremia, hypercalcemia, and uremia. Metabolic abnormalities can also lead to the development of organic mental syndromes that can further decrease oral intake. Many drugs, such as the narcotic analgesics and the theophylline derivatives, can cause severe nausea. If left untreated, nausea and vomiting can lead to anorexia. Finally, psychological and psychiatric factors also play a role in the etiology of anorexia and weight loss in terminally ill patients. Among the most frequent of such causes are anxiety, depression, and conditioned food aversions (Lesko 1989).

The treatment of anorexia and weight loss begins with the identification and correction of its reversible causes. For example, when uncontrolled opioid-induced nausea is identified as a key factor in a patient's inability to eat, adding an antiemetic may completely control the subsequent anorexia. Once specific causes have been ruled out or corrected, subsequent treatment relies on environmental manipulations (Levy and Catalano 1985). Frequent administration of favorite foods, nutritional supplements, and fluids can reverse weight loss. Pharmacological stimulation of appetite is an area of current interest and research investigation. (For a detailed discussion, see Chapter 4.) Corticosteroids such as prednisone 5–10 mg tid, methylprednisolone 8–16 mg tid, or dexamethasone 2–4 mg po tid have been reported to increase appetite as well as produce a sense of well-being in cachectic and anorexic patients with advanced cancer (Hanks et al. 1983). Cyproheptadine hydrochloride (Periactin) is an antiserotonin agent, commonly used to treat pruritus, that has been found to cause weight gain and appetite stimulation when is given in doses of 4 mg tid 30 minutes before meals (Dombrowski 1982).

Megestrol acetate (Megace), which is a progestational agent used in the treatment of breast cancer, has been showed to promote weight gain and increase appetite in terminally ill cancer patients when given in a regimen starting with 20 mg po tid, up to 160 mg/day (Tchekmedyian et al. 1986). In a randomized, double-blind, placebo-controlled trial (Loprinzi et al. 1990), cancer patients with anorexia and cachexia experienced significant ($P<.003$) appetite stimulation and weight gain on megestrol acetate 800 mg/day (16% of 67 patients gained 15 lb or more).

When poor appetite is a symptom of underlying major depression or significant anxiety, psychopharmacological interventions with antidepressants (tricyclics or psychostimulants) and anxiolytics are indicated. Conditioned nausea and vomiting are often quite responsive to relaxation training and other behavioral techniques (Redd 1989). These interventions can be used even by patients with advanced disease if their sensorium is clear and they are capable of concentrating.

Mouth Discomfort

Pain and discomfort of the oral cavity are among the most common difficulties that affect nutritional intake and quality of life in patients with advanced cancer (DeConno et al. 1989; Twycross and Lack 1986). In addition to profoundly diminishing the innate pleasures of eating and drinking, oral lesions can compromise verbal communication. The psychological sequelae of being unable to speak clearly include a sense of isolation, frustration, and/or demoralization. Oral pain and discomfort, like anorexia, weight loss, and pain, comprise a multifactorial problem. Among the many causes of oral pain are infections, neutropenic ulcers, drug-induced stomatitis, and dry mouth.

Infections of the oral cavity can be fungal, viral, or bacterial in nature and can occur either singly or in combination. Oral candidiasis is the most common infection and is treated with clotrimazole (Mycelex Troches 10 mg) dissolved in the mouth four to five times a day. Ketoconazole (Nizoral) 200 mg po bid is also helpful. In more severe cases, amphotericin B 10–20 mg iv daily for 5–7 days is indicated. Among the viral infections of the oral cavity, herpes simplex is the most common. Herpes simplex is treated with acyclovir 200 mg po every 4 hours for 5–7 days. Occasionally, with disseminated herpes, intravenous acyclovir is necessary. The clinician should be aware that delirium is a common complication of intravenous acyclovir. Finally, poor oral hygiene and neutropenia may predispose the patient to bacterial infections.

A painful mouth can also be caused by chemotherapy-induced stomatitis, neutropenic ulcers, or fungating lesions. Such problems require an approach that combines good mouth care and aggressive pain control. The judicious use of adequate amounts of narcotic analgesics are essential. It is also important to note that the appearance of the lesion is not always an accurate measure of how painful it is experienced by the patient. Some healing lesions are still quite painful. Hypnosis and relaxation interventions can be helpful in the management of painful stomatitis experienced during bone-marrow transplantation. Good mouth care is generally helpful in dealing with oral pain. Glyoxide rinses (conthiacy hydroxen penexide, benzocaine, and flavoring), chlorhexidine (Peridex), or 1% povidone-iodine (Betadine)-specific oral products can be helpful along with gentle mechanical cleansing. Corticosteroids applied as creams can also be soothing. Oral local anesthetics are probably most helpful, particularly viscous xylocaine 2% solution (5–10 ml or 10% oral spray every 3 hours) or choline salicylate paste (applied every 3–4 hours).

Dry mouth can be caused by radiotherapy to the oral cavity and dehydration and is also a common side effect of many medications (Deconno et al 1989; Nally 1989). When severe, dry mouth can cause discomfort, trouble talking or swallowing, and taste alteration. Oral swishing with a solution of 2% citric acid or pilocarpine can reduce discomfort. Artificial saliva (Salivart, as metered oral spray) or carboxymethylcellulose (Xerolube, 5 ml) can be given as needed. When dehydration is thought to be the cause of dry mouth, it should, where possible, be corrected. Tricyclics, phenothiazines, and narcotic analgesics can all cause or exacerbate dry mouth. Bearing this in mind, the psychiatric consultant can prescribe psychotropics with lower-anticholinergic activity or reduce the dosages of highly anticholinergic medications to minimize contributing to this problem.

Taste Alteration

Taste alteration is another oral complication of advanced cancer (DeConno et al. 1989). Although it is infrequently reported by patients in a spontaneous fashion, it is a common cause of loss of pleasure in eating and can lead to anorexia. The effects of cancer on taste are incompletely understood. Some potential causes of taste alteration include direct effects of oral cancers on the mouth and tongue, brain lesions or treatment-related injuries to the nervous system, side effects of radiotherapy and chemotherapy, malnutrition, and metabolic disturbances. Of interest, plasma zinc levels are low in certain cancers, and zinc deficiency has been suggested as a factor in taste alteration. Some tips for restoring enjoyment of food and decreasing anorexia among patients with altered taste are 1) serve food hot and presented attractively, 2) serve foods with strong odors (lemon and vinegar may help), 3) use therapies that maintain or increase salivation, 4) optimize oral hygiene, and 5) eliminate drugs that may be causing this symptom.

Dysphagia

Dysphagia (difficulty swallowing) and odynophagia (pain on swallowing) have causes and treatments similar to those of the oral complications described above (Levy and Catalano 1985). Some unusual causes of dysphagia include obstruction of the esophagus due to external compression by mediastinal tumor or lymphadenopathy. Radiation-induced stricture of the esophagus can also occur. General measures to deal with dysphagia include the use of soft, pureed, or liquid diets, as well as the avoidance of oral medications. Bypassing the oral route through the use of gastrostomy feeding tubes can be helpful, as can the use of parenteral hyperalimentation. Occasionally the palliative use of chemotherapy or radiation to shrink a compressing mediastinal mass is warranted. Viscous lidocaine solution 2% (5–10 ml) before meals is helpful with odynophagia. Antacids or histamine receptor blockers such as cimetidine (300 mg po every 6 hours) or ranitidine (150 mg po every 12 hours) are indicated for reflux esophagitis. Fungal esophagitis is treated with oral or systemic antifungals as discussed above.

Nausea and Vomiting

Approximately 50% of patients with advanced cancer experience nausea and vomiting during the course of their illness (Barnes 1988; Levy and Catalano 1985). Common causes of nausea and vomiting in cancer patients include chemotherapy, radiation, medications, toxins, metabolic derangements, and obstruction of the gastrointestinal tract. Emesis occurs as a result of stimulation of the vomiting center in the medullary reticular formation. This vomiting center lies structurally close to the chemoreceptor trigger zone (CTZ) in the area postrema of the fourth ventricle. Vomiting induced by radiation, antineoplastic therapies, and other drugs is mediated through the CTZ, which stimulates the vomiting center. The vomiting center can be stimulated through a variety of routes including the CTZ and afferents coming from the cerebral cortex, gastrointestinal tract, heart, and the vestibular system.

Chemotherapy is a common cause of nausea and vomiting in cancer patients. There is great variability in the emetogenic properties of the various cytotoxic agents; however, cisplatin, dacarbazine, actinomycin D, cyclophosphamide, and nitrogen mustard have such high emetic potential that virtually all patients can be expected to experience significant nausea and vomiting (Kris and Gralla 1990). A variety of medications used in the cancer setting can cause nausea and vomiting including the narcotic analgesics, estrogens, aspirin, NSAIDs, steroids, digitalis, and theophylline. Many of these drugs cause nausea by inducing a gastritis or promoting gastric stasis.

Metabolic disturbances such as hypercalcemia and hypomagnesemia can also cause nausea and vomiting. Uremia resulting from renal or hepatic failure is often a terminal event in the far-advanced cancer patient and is frequently accompanied by nausea and vomiting. Mechanical obstruction of the intestinal tract due to advanced ovarian or colonic cancers can lead to nausea and vomiting that can be difficult to manage. Increased intracranial pressure due to central nervous system spread or primary brain cancers are well-known, but infrequent, causes of intractable nausea.

Given the numerous possible etiologies of nausea and vomiting in cancer patients with advanced disease, appropriate treatment is predicated on a careful assessment. Choice of specific therapy will depend on the etiology of the nausea and vomiting as well as on the degree to which aggressive diagnostics or treatment is warranted. For example, patients with increased brain metastases would benefit most from administration of high-dose corticosteroids. Patients with intractable vomiting due to mechanical obstruction of the intestinal tract often respond best to surgical interventions such as diverting procedures that can be done with minimal invasiveness or to start courses of steroid therapy to decrease inflammation and swelling. In general, the approach to the control of emesis is symptomatic, using antiemetic drugs. In the setting of terminal illness, in which comfort is the goal of therapy, it is sometimes quite difficult to determine how much investigation of the etiology of nausea and vomiting is optimal. Certainly a blood test to determine if the patient is hypercalcemic or uremic is helpful in guiding therapy and produces little discomfort. In addition, one cannot underestimate the helpfulness of a simple physical examination of the patient and a thoughtful history in determining the cause of emesis.

Antiemetic drugs are the mainstay of managing nausea and vomiting in cancer patients with advanced disease. Dopamine antagonists (e.g., metoclopramide, haloperidol, droperidol, and prochlorperazine), glucocorticoids (e.g., dexamethasone and methylprednisolone), and benzodiazepines (e.g., lorazepam) are the most effective antiemetics available and are used either alone or in combination (Barnes 1988; Kris and Gralla 1990).

Metoclopramide is an effective antiemetic in cancer patients undergoing chemotherapy because it is a potent antagonist of central dopamine receptors in the CTZ. Because of their dopamine-blocking properties, metoclopramide and other dopamine-antagonists can cause extrapyramidal reactions and even tardive dyskinesia when used in high dosages (Breitbart 1986). Lorazepam, a benzodiazepine, is a useful antiemetic, especially in combination with other agents, and is characterized by a unique ability to induce anxiolysis, anterograde amnesia, and a dampening response of the vomiting center (Kearsley et al. 1989). The main adverse effects of lorazepam are sedation and the amnestic properties that some patients actually find quite beneficial. Antihistaminic agents, anticholinergic drugs, marijuana, and the synthetic cannabinoids (e.g., nabilone) have also been used, but have limited efficacy. Δ^9-tetrahydrocannabinol (THC), like the phenothiazines, has antiemetic efficacy greater than placebo, but is less potent than other available agents (e.g., metoclopramide, dexamethasone, and lorazepam) and is associated with a high number of adverse reactions including paranoid ideation (Frytak et al. 1979). New research suggests that serotonin may be a mediator of nausea and emesis induced by chemotherapy. Ondansetron is a selective antagonist of serotonin, subtype 3 (S3), receptors and has been demonstrated to be an effective

Table 8–9.   Dosages and routes of antiemetic agents

Antiemetic agent (by class)	Dosage	Route
Dopamine antagonists		
Metoclopramide	1–3 mg/kg	Every 2–3 hours iv
	10–20 mg	Every 6 hours po
Haloperidol	1–2 mg	Every 2–6 hours po
	1–2 mg	Every 2–6 hours iv, sc
Prochlorperazine	5–10 mg	Every 2–4 hours po
	25 mg	Every 4–6 hours pr
	10–15 mg	Every 2–4 hours im
	10–20 mg	Every 3–6 hours iv
Chlorpromazine	25–50 mg	Every 3–6 hours po
	12.5–25 mg	Every 4–6 hours im
	12.5–25 mg	Every 4–6 hours iv
Serotonin antagonists		
Ondansetron	0.15 mg/kg	Every 1.5–3.5 hours iv
Corticosteroids		
Dexamethasone	4–16 mg	Daily po, iv or every 4–6 hours po, iv
Methylprednisolone	250–500 mg	Daily iv or every 4–6 hours iv
Benzodiazepines		
Lorazepam	1–2 mg	Every 2–6 hours po, iv
Cannabinoids		
Δ^9-tetrahydrocannabinol (THC)	5–10 mg/m^2	Every 3–4 hours po

Note.   po = oral; iv = intravenous; im = intramuscular; sc = subcutaneous; pr = per rectum.

antiemetic when used to treat cisplatin-induced nausea and vomiting (Cubeddu et al. 1990).

When administering antiemetic drugs, the oral route is often possible; however, many of these drugs can be given intravenously, intramuscularly, or by rectal suppository when the oral route is unavailable. Table 8–9 lists frequently used antiemetic agents and their dosage regimens.

Constipation and Bowel Obstruction

Constipation is another common and distressing problem in patients with advanced cancer (Levy and Catalano 1985; Portenoy 1987; Twycross and Lack 1990a). Inactivity, poor fluid intake, generalized weakness, narcotic analgesics, metabolic abnormalities, and anticholinergic side effects of drugs can all contribute to constipation. When possible, the best treatment for constipation is prophylactic. Patients should be encouraged to increase fluid and dietary fiber intake, as well as to increase their activity and ambulate. Patients who are to receive narcotic opioid analgesics should be prophylactically treated with stool softeners and laxatives before constipation develops. Senna derivatives are effective because they contain a stool softener and bowel stimulant. Other laxatives that are helpful in avoiding constipation with analgesics include casanthranol (Peri-Colace), psyllium (Metamucil), and lactulose (Cephulac). The elimination of constipating anticholinergic drugs when possible is essential.

Bowel obstruction can occur as a result of peritoneal carcinomatosis, postsurgical or postradiation adhesions or strictures, or chemotherapy-induced paralytic ileus. Signs and symptoms of bowel obstruction include abdominal pain, tenderness, distension, constipation, overflow diarrhea, air-fluid level on X ray, visible peristalsis, and tinkling bowel sounds. In the management of bowel obstruction in dying patients, the goal is to treat the symptoms of obstruction without having to resort to surgery. The pain and colic due to peristalsis in the face of obstruction is most problematic and is best managed through the use of antiperistaltic and antidiarrheal agents. Narcotic analgesics such as morphine (5–10 mg every 4 hours) or hydromorphone (1–4 mg every 4 hours) are helpful. Transdermal scopolamine, atropine, or diphenoxylate with atropine (Lomotil 2 tablets qid) help diminish peristalsis. Antiemetics given either orally, parenterally, or rectally, as well as corticosteroids, are useful in diminishing nausea and vomiting second-ary to obstruction.

The following case example illustrates the psychiatric importance of aggressive management of gastrointestinal and other physical symptoms in the patient with terminal illness:

Case 6

A psychiatric consultation was requested for Ms. V, a 43-year-old divorced woman with advanced gastric cancer, to rule out depression. She had been initially diagnosed a year earlier and had undergone a subtotal gastrectomy and systemic chemotherapy. Having apparently suffered an anxious period of adjustment, she had been prescribed lorazepam 0.5 mg prn bid by her surgeon. She had moved in with her mother during her convalescence and had benefited from group and supportive individual psychotherapy. However, she had recently en-countered pain and anorexia, and evaluation revealed recurrent cancer. Ms. V was admitted to the hospital for evaluation of suitability for experimental chemotherapy, but her condition soon deteriorated. She underwent surgery and was left with a jejunostomy.

Ms. V withdrew into her room and canceled visits from her social worker-therapist and group members. She described to the consultant that although these people had been helpful she was now "too de-pressed" to benefit from them. In the interview, she revealed that she had been in pain since her surgery and that this had led to thoughts about wanting to die. She had pain at the J-tube site and constant abdominal cramping and nausea, unrelieved by morphine, metoclo-pramide, and prochlorperazine. Ms. V also complained of anxiety (unrelieved by infrequent as-needed doses of lorazepam), which on further assessment was more accurately diagnosed as akathisia caused by antiemetics. She also revealed that 3 days earlier she had suffered delusions and hallucinations during the night, which she had not reported to staff for fear that they would think that she was "crazy." Ms. V was mildly sedated but oriented and nonpsychotic during the interview. Her mood was slightly depressed, and, al-though she had had thoughts of dying, she denied helplessness or hopelessness.

The consultant diagnosed akathisia, uncontrolled pain and nausea, and delirium and made several recommendations. Ms. V was placed on a standing dose of lorazepam 0.5 mg every 4 hours, neuroleptic antiemetics were discontinued, and a pain service consultant discontinued her morphine and started a shorter-acting opioid analgesic (Dilaudid). Over the next 2 days, the dosages of the analgesic and anxiolytic were titrated. The third day after the consultation, Ms. V stated she felt "normal again" and resumed contact with her psychosocial supports. There was no evidence of an independent mood disorder after the relief of her physical symptoms.

Hiccups

Hiccups are involuntary contractions of the diaphragm. Common causes of hiccups in cancer patients include general toxic conditions such as uremia or hepatic encephalopathy, diaphragmatic irritation due to gastric distension, subphrenic abscesses, central nervous system metastases, or phrenic nerve irritation. Intractable hiccups can be exhausting and distressing. A variety of physical measures are helpful in managing hiccups and gastric distension that may be contributing to the problem. Nasogastric tube insertion and the use of antifoaming agents (simethicone) and/or antacids are helpful in reducing gaseous distension. Pharyngeal vagal stimulation using either swallowed ice water, granulated sugar, or a nasogastric catheter often results in rapid cessation of hiccups. Pharmacological management of intractable hiccups (Levy and Catalano 1985) includes:

1. Chlorpromazine—25–50 mg po or slow intravenous infusion every 6 hours
2. Haloperidol—3–5 mg po or intravenously every 4–6 hours
3. Metoclopramide—10–20 mg po every 4–6 hours
4. Carbamazepine—100–200 mg every 8 hours
5. Phenytoin—100 mg qid (carbamazepine and phenytoin are helpful especially if hiccups are due to a central nervous system lesion)
6. Quinidine—200 mg every 6 hours
7. Dexamethasone—4–8 mg po every 3–4 hours (especially with hepatomegaly)
8. Nifedipine—10–20 mg po every 8 hours (Mukhopadhyay et al. 1986)

Dyspnea

Breathlessness (dyspnea) is a common and distressing symptom in the terminally ill patient population (Fishbein et al. 1989). Primary lung cancers, the most frequent causes of death in both men and women, commonly cause dyspnea (Twycross and Lack 1990b). Pulmonary metastases are extremely common (almost one-third of cancer patients have pulmonary metastases at autopsy), and these are another frequent cause of shortness of breath. Other causes of dyspnea include pleural effusion, anemia, congestive heart failure, pneumonia, bronchospasm, and treatment-related lung damage (from chemotherapy and/or radiotherapy). When breathlessness develops acutely, non–cancer-related disease processes must be considered (i.e., myocardial infarction or angina, cardiac dysrhythmias, and pulmonary embolism). Specific diagnoses demand specific medical therapies, such as antibiotics for pneumonia or diuretics for congestive heart failure.

After specific diagnoses and complications have been treated or ruled out, the physician is often left with a patient who remains short of breath and anxious. This anxiety is often referred to as "air hunger" and can be overwhelming to patient, family, and staff. When possible, it can be helpful to modify the disease process in the lung causing dyspnea through the use of palliative radiation or thoracentesis to remove fluid. Some general measures to reduce dyspnea include supplementary oxygen (intranasally), relaxation exercises, and manipulation of the environment to induce relaxation. Morphine, anxiolytics, anticholinergic agents, bronchodilators, and steroids all play a role in the pharmacological management of dyspnea. Morphine can be given orally or intravenously 2.5–5 mg qid as needed or as a continuous intravenous infusion starting with 1–3 mg/hour and titrated up toward a level providing comfort (Twycross and Lack 1990b). Lorazepam 0.5–2 mg po or iv every 4 hours can be quite effective, as can midazolam used as a continuous infusion.

Cough

A persistent cough is yet another respiratory symptom that can cause considerable physical and psychological distress (Levy and Catalano 1985). Coughing can result in sleeplessness, pain, and nausea and vomiting. Reversible pulmonary causes of persistent cough are the same as discussed in the section on dyspnea above. Persistent cough can be controlled with narcotic analgesics, which are central nervous system cough suppressants. Morphine 5 mg every 4 hours or codeine 15–30 mg every 4 hours is used to suppress cough. Meperidine has little if any antitussive potency. Other antitussives include scopolamine, atropine, and inhaled bupivacaine 0.25%. Steroids, humidifiers, and artificial saliva are sometimes helpful in controlling cough.

Death Rattle

Cancer patients, with pulmonary involvement of their disease, frequently have difficulty clearing the large airway secretions that accumulate. A disheartening and frightening sound, the so-called death rattle, that results is not limited to dying patients, although it is most frequently encountered in terminal stages of disease. This sound can be distressing for staff, family, and other patients. The patient in this advanced state is usually obtunded. Thus it is often helpful and comforting to describe to family members just what the patient's level of awareness is and to explain that there is little likelihood that the patient is suffering. The treatment of this highly symbolic symptom includes postural drainage through physiotherapy and/or the topical administration of a scopolamine patch. Scopolamine both dries accumulated secretions and induces relaxation of smooth bronchial musculature. Atropine is also used quite frequently, although its tendency to precipitate central nervous system excitation renders scopolamine preferable in many cases (Twycross and Lack 1990b).

Urinary Symptoms

Retention of urine can lead to urinary tract infection and abdominal pain or discomfort. Severe urinary retention can precipitate renal failure. Urinary symptoms can arise from multiple etiologies; thus they too require careful evaluation and assessment before treatment. Among the many possible causes of urinary retention in patients with advanced cancer are 1) bladder outlet obstruction from tumor extension, 2) nonmalignant obstruction (stricture and prostatic hypertrophy), 3) neurogenic bladder (spinal cord compression and cerebral tumor), and 4) medication reactions (anticholinergics, sympathomimetics, antipsychotics, and tricyclic antidepressants). Treatment with bethanechol (10–30 mg po three to four times a day) may be effective for some patients, though most will require insertion of a Foley catheter.

Urinary frequency and incontinence are also common symptoms that can be particularly distressing to patients. Among the leading causes of these problems are 1) metabolic abnormalities (hypercalcemia, diabetes mellitus, and diabetes insipidus), 2) urinary tract infections, 3) radiation effects, 4) neurological lesions, and 5) pelvic involvement of disease. The treatment of urinary frequency and incontinence begins with aggressive medical management. For example, diabetes should be treated with oral hypoglycemics or insulin. When possible, hypercalcemia should similarly be corrected. Urinary tract infections require antibiotic therapy. Finally, acute spinal cord compression can present with urinary incontinence. When acute spinal cord compression is suspected, urgent myelography and subsequent therapy with steroids, radiotherapy, or decompression laminectomy may be indicated (Levy and Catalano 1985). When urinary incontinence requires the chronic use of an indwelling catheter, it is helpful to use ascorbic acid, 100 mg po qid or a urinary antiseptic such as methenamine hippurate (1 g po tid) to minimize the incidence of urinary tract infection.

Cutaneous Symptoms

Pruritus, or generalized itching, can cause anxiety, skin excoriation, and skin infection. Common causes of pruritus in terminal cancer patients include dry skin, obstructive jaundice, uremia, drug allergy, and malignancy. Management begins with the elimination of potential irritants (Twycross and Lack 1990c). For example, a careful review of medicines may lead to the discovery of a new agent that is causing the syndrome. Topical creams, such as lanolin or 1% hydrocortisone, applied three to four times a day are often helpful.

Systemic antihistamines are effective for pruritus, although they have unfortunate side effect profiles for this population. Among these side effects, sedation, dry mouth, and decreased bowel motility are all too frequent and can serve to exacerbate existing problems. Cyproheptadine, a serotonin antagonist and antihistamine, can be quite a useful alternative. Hydroxyzine is an effective treatment in doses of 25–60 mg every 6–8 hours. In addition, diligent skin care is critical in the management of pruritus. Such care includes avoiding the use of swabs, scratching, and overheating or perspiring. Other skin complications encountered by patients with advanced cancer are decubitus ulcers and fungating lesions. (A detailed description of these symptoms is beyond the scope of this chapter. For reviews, see Renler and Cooney 1980 and Foltz 1980.)

Asthenia

Asthenia is defined as generalized weakness and physical or mental fatigue. Studies (e.g., Bruera and MacDonald 1988) suggest that as many as two-thirds of patients with advanced cancer complain of weakness. Unfortunately, a treatable cause of asthenia will be identified and corrected in only a minority of cases. The role of psychiatric factors in the presentation of asthenia in dying cancer patients is small in comparison with that of physical factors. However, psychiatric factors are probably enlisted too often by frustrated staff who have seen a number of treatments fail and then view patients' continuing malaise as a sign of depression. More likely, the cause of asthenia arises from 1) malnutrition, 2) infection, 3) profound anemia, 4) metabolic abnormalities, and/or 5) medication reactions. Chemotherapeutic agents and radiotherapy are frequently used as palliative therapies in patients with advanced cancer. Both can cause significant weakness that may resolve after treatment is completed.

The psychological and psychiatric treatment of asthenic patients includes patient and family education (i.e., especially to address the nonpsychological nature of the problem in many cases). An ongoing supportive relationship that permits patients to express fears and concerns about the meaning of continued weakness and to address distorted ideas that they may have about its prognostic significance is critically important (Bruera and MacDonald 1988). We have encountered several patients who were suffering with temporary asthenia from chemotherapy or radiotherapy who felt that their weakness was a sign of imminent death. The literature in support of the pharmacotherapy of asthenia in cancer patients is largely anecdotal. Some patients respond to steroids (e.g., methylprednisolone 15–30 mg daily) with improvement in mood, appetite, and physical well-being. Unfortunately, this response tends to be fleeting. Also problematic is the fact that prolonged use of steroids can exacerbate weakness by causing proximal myopathy. Steroids have several other potentially distressing adverse effects including severe psychiatric syndromes such as organic mood syndromes and delirium. Psychostimulants have been used in the treatment of asthenia with mixed results. However, certain patients do respond well to amphetamine, methylphenidate, or pemoline, and it has been our practice to use stimulants not only for depressive syndromes but for the asthenia and weakness syndrome as well.

Summary

Palliative care of terminally ill or dying cancer patients has become an important part of cancer treatment in general. The role of the psychiatrist or other mental health professional in the care of terminally ill or dying patients is critical to both adequate symptom control and integration of the physical, psychological, and spiritual dimensions of human experience in the last weeks of life. To be most effective in this role, the psychiatrist must not only have specialized knowledge of the psychiatric complications of terminal illness, but must also be familiar with the common physical symptoms that plague the patient with advanced cancer and contribute so dramatically to suffering.

References

Achte KA, Vanhkouen ML: Cancer and the psyche. Omega 2:46–56, 1971

Adams F, Fernandez F, Andersson BS: Emergency pharmacotherapy of delirium in the critically ill cancer patient. Psychosomatics 27:33–37, 1986

American Psychiatric Association: Diagnostic and Statistical Manual of Mental Disorders, 3rd Edition. Washington, DC, American Psychiatric Association, 1980

Barnes M: Nausea and vomiting in the patient with advanced cancer. Journal of Pain and Symptom Management 3:81–85, 1988

Beaver WT, Feise E: Comparison of the analgesic effects of morphine hydroxyzine and their combination in patients with post-operative pain, in Proceedings of the First World Congress on Pain: Advances in Pain Research. Edited by Bonica JJ. New York, Raven, 1976, pp 553–557

Beaver WT, Wallenstein SM, Houde RW, et al: A comparison of the analgesic effects of methotrimeprazine and morphine in patients with cancer. Clin Pharmacol Ther 17:276–291, 1966

Beck AT, Kovacs M, Weissman A: Hopelessness and suicidal behavior: an overview. JAMA 234:1146–1149, 1975

Bolund C: Suicide and cancer, I: demographic and social characteristics of cancer patients who committed suicide in Sweden, 1973–1976. Journal of Psychosocial Oncology 3:17–30, 1985a

Bolund C: Suicide and cancer, II: medical and care factors in suicides by cancer patients in Sweden, 1973–1976. J Psychosoc Oncol 3:31–52, 1985b

Breitbart W: Tardive dyskinesia associated with high-dose intravenous metaclopramide (letter). N Engl J Med 315:518, 1986

Breitbart W: Suicide in cancer patients. Oncology 1:49–54, 1987

Breitbart W: Psychiatric management of cancer pain. Cancer 63:2336–2342,

1989

Breitbart W: Cancer pain and suicide, in Advances in Pain Research and Therapy, Vol 16. Edited by Foley KM, Bonica JJ, Ventafridda V. New York, Raven, 1990, pp 399–411

Breitbart W, Holland J: Psychiatric Aspects of Cancer Pain, in Advances in Pain Research and Therapy, Vol 16. Edited by Foley KM, Bonica JJ, Ventafridda V. New York, Raven, 1990, pp 73–87

Brodie G: Indomethacin and bone pain (letter). Lancet 2:1160, 1974

Brown JH, Henteleff P, Barakat S, et al: Is it normal for terminally ill patients to desire death? Am J Psychiatry 143:208–211, 1986

Bruera E: Symptom control in patients with cancer. Journal of Psychosocial Oncology 8:47–73, 1990

Bruera E, MacDonald N: Asthenia in patients with advanced cancer. Journal of Pain and Symptom Management 3:9–14, 1988

Bruera E, Chadwick S, Brennels C, et al: Methylphenidate associated with narcotics for the treatment of cancer pain. Cancer Treatment Reports 71:67–70, 1987

Bruera E, Brenneis C, Paterson AH, et al: Use of methylphenidate as an adjuvant to narcotic analgesics in patients with advanced cancer. Journal of Pain and Symptom Management 4:3–6, 1989

Bukberg J, Penman D, Holland J: Depression in hospitalized cancer patients. Psychosom Med 46:199–212, 1984

Cassem NH: The dying patient, in Massachusetts General Hospital Handbook of General Hospital Psychiatry, 2nd Edition. Edited by Hackett TP, Cassem NH. Littleton, MA, PSG Publishing, 1987, pp 332–352

Ciraulo DA, Shader RI: Fluoxetine drug-drug interactions, I: antidepressants and antipsychotics. J Clin Psychopharmacol 10:48–50, 1990

Coyle N, Adelhardt J, Foley KM, et al: Character of terminal illness in the advanced cancer patient: pain and other symptoms during the last four weeks of life. Journal of Pain and Symptom Management 5:83–93, 1990

Cubeddu LX, Hoffmann IS, Fuenmayor NT, et al: Efficacy of odansetron (GR 38032F) and the role of serotonin in cisplatin-induced nausea and vomiting. N Engl J Med 322:810–816,1990

DeConno F, Ripamonti C, Sbanotto A, et al: Oral complications in patients with advanced cancer. Journal of Pain and Symptom Management 4:20–30, 1989

Derogatis LR, Morrow GR, Fetting J, et al: The prevalence of psychiatric disorders among cancer patients. JAMA 249:715–757, 1983

Dombrowski SR: Cyproheptadine for producing weight gain in children and adults. Hospital Formulary 17:1503–1512, 1982

Dubovsky SL: Averting suicide in terminally ill patients. Psychosomatics 19:113–115, 1978

Elliott K, Foley KM: Neurologic pain syndromes in patients with cancer, in Pain

Mechanisms and Syndromes, Neurologic Clinics. Edited by Portenoy RK. Philadelphia, PA, WB Saunders, 1989, pp 333–360

Elliott K, Foley KM: Pain syndromes in the cancer patient. Journal of Psychosocial Oncology 8:11–45, 1990

Endicott J: Measurement of depression in patients with cancer. Cancer 53:2243–2248, 1984

Farberow NL, Schneidman ES, Leonard VV: Suicide Among General Medical and Surgical Hospital Patients With Malignant Neoplasm: Medical Bulletin 9. Washington, DC, U.S. Veterans Administration, 1963

Farberow NL, Ganzler S, Cuter F, et al: An eight-year survey of hospital suicides. Suicide Life Threat Behav 1:184–201, 1971

Fernandez F, Adams F, Holmes VF, et al: Methylphenidate for depressive disorders in cancer patients. Psychosomatics 28:455–461, 1987

Fishbein D, Kearson C, Killian KJ: An approach to dyspnea in cancer patients. Journal of Pain and Symptom Management 4:76–81, 1989

Fishman B, Pasternak S, Wallenstein SL, et al: The Memorial Pain Assessment Card: a valid instrument for the evaluation of cancer pain. Cancer 60:1151–1158, 1987

Foley KM: Pain syndromes in patients with cancer, in Advances in Pain Research and Therapy, Vol 2. Edited by Bonica JJ, Ventafridda V. New York, Raven, 1979, pp 59–75

Foley KM: The treatment of cancer pain. N Engl J Med 313:84–95, 1985

Foley KM: Pain syndromes in patients with cancer, in Cancer Pain: Medical Clinics of North America. Edited by Payne R, Foley KM. Philadelphia, PA, WB Saunders, 1987, pp 169–184

Foley KM, Inturrisi CE: Analgesic drug therapy in cancer pain: principles and practice, in Cancer Pain: Medical Clinics of North America. Edited by Payne R, Foley KM. Philadelphia, PA, WB Saunders, 1987, pp 207–232

Foltz AT: Nursing care of ulcerating metastatic lesions. Oncology Nursing Forum 7:8–13, 1980

Fox BH, Stanek EJ, Boyd SC, et al: Suicide rates among cancer patients in Connecticut. Journal of Chronic Diseases 35:85–100, 1982

Frytak S, Moertel CG, O'Fallon JR: Delta-9-tetrahydrocannabinol as an antiemetic for patients receiving chemotherapy. Ann Intern Med 91:825–830, 1979

Guze S, Robins E: Suicide and primary affective disorders. Br J Psychiatry 117:437–438, 1970

Hanks GW, Trueman T, Twycross EG: Corticosteroids in terminal cancer: a prospective analgesic of current practice. Postgrad Med J 59:28–32, 1983

Helig S: The San Francisco Medical Society euthanasia survey: results and analysis. San Francisco Medicine 61:24–34, 1988

Holland JC: Psychological aspects of cancer, in Cancer Medicine, 2nd Edition.

Edited by Holland JF, Frei E. Philadelphia, PA, Lea & Febiger, 1982, pp 1175–1205

Holland JC: Anxiety and cancer: the patient and the family. J Clin Psychiatry 50:20–25, 1989

Hollister LE: Pharmacotherapeutic considerations in anxiety disorders. J Clin Psychiatry 47:33–36, 1986

Inturrisi C: Management of cancer pain. Cancer 63:2308–2326, 1989

Kaiko R, Foley K, Grabinski P, et al: Central nervous system excitatory effects of meperidine in cancer patients. Ann Neurol 13:180–183, 1983

Kantor TG: Peripherally acting analgesics, in Analgesics: Neurochemical, Behavioral, and Clinical Perspectives. Edited by Kuhar M, Pasternak G. New York, Raven, 1984, pp 289–313

Kearsley JH, Williams AN, Flumara AM: Antiemetic superiority of lorazepam over oxazepam and methylprednisolone as premedicants for patients receiving cisplatin-containing chemotherapy. Cancer 64:1595–1599, 1989

Kovacs M, Beck AT, Weissman A: Hopelessness: an indication of suicidal risk. Suicide 5:98–103, 1975

Kris MG, Gralla RJ: Management of vomiting caused by anticancer drugs, in Advances in Pain Research and Therapy, Vol 16. Edited by Foley KM, Bonica JJ, Ventafridda V. New York, Raven Press, 1990, pp 337–344

Lesko L: Anorexia, in Handbook of Psychooncology: Psychological Care of the Patient With Cancer. Edited by Holland JC, Rowland JH. New York, Oxford University Press, 1989, pp 434–443

Lesko L, Holland JC: Psychosocial complications of leukemia, in Leukemia, 5th Edition. Edited by Henderson ES, Lister TA. Philadelphia, PA, WB Saunders, 1989, pp 769–794

Levine PM, Silberfarb PM, Lipowski ZJ: Mental disorders in cancer patients. Cancer 42:1385–1390, 1978

Levy M, Catalano R: Control of common physical symptoms other than pain in patients with terminal disease. Semin Oncol 12:411–430, 1985

Liebowitz MR: Imipramine in the treatment of panic disorder and its complications. Psychiatr Clin North Am 8:37–47, 1985

Loprinzi CL, Ellison NM, Schaid DJ, et al: Controlled trial of megestrol acetate for the treatment of cancer anorexia and cachexia. J Natl Cancer Inst 82:1127–1132, 1990

Louhivuori KA, Hakama J: Risk of suicide among cancer patients. Am J Epidemiol 109:59–65, 1979

Macaluso C, Weinberg D, Foley KM: Opioid abuse and misuse in a cancer pain population (abstract). Journal of Pain and Symptom Management 3:54, 1988

Marks RM, Sachar EJ: Undertreatment of medical inpatients with narcotic analgesics. Ann Intern Med 78:173–181, 1973

Massie MJ: Anxiety, panic and phobias, in Handbook of Psychooncology: Psychological Care of the Patient With Cancer. Edited by Holland JC, Rowland JH. New York, Oxford University Press, 1989, pp 300–309

Massie MJ, Holland JC: Diagnosis and treatment of depression in the cancer patient. J Clin Psychiatry 42:25–28, 1984

Massie MJ, Holland JC: The cancer patient with pain: psychiatric complications and their management. Med Clin North Am 71:243–257, 1987

Massie MJ, Gorzynski JG, Mastrovito RC, et al: The diagnosis of depression in hospitalized patients. Proceedings of the American Association of Cancer Research/American Society of Clinical Oncology 20:432–440, 1979

Massie MJ, Holland JC, Glass E: Delirium in terminally ill cancer patients. Am J Psychiatry 140:1048–1050, 1983

McKegney PP, Lange P: The decision to no longer live on chronic hemodialysis. Am J Psychiatry 128:47–55, 1971

Mukhopadhyay P, Osman MR, Wajima T, et al: Nifedipine for intractable hiccups (letter). N Engl J Med 314:1256, 1986

Murphy GE: Suicide and attempted suicide. Hosp Pract 12:78–81, 1977

Murray GB: Confusion, delirium, and dementia, in Massachusetts General Hospital Handbook of General Hospital Psychiatry, 2nd Edition. Edited by Hackett TP, Cassem NH. Littleton, MA, PSG Publishing Company, 1987, pp 84–115

Nally F: Xerostomia, in Symptom Control. Edited by Walsh TD. Boston, MA, Blackwell Scientific, 1989, pp 430–440

Pearson HJ: Interaction of fluoxetine with carbamazepine (letter). J Clin Psychiatry 51:126, 1990

Plumb MM, Holland JC: Comparative studies of psychological function in patients with advanced cancer. Psychosom Med 39:264–276, 1977

Portenoy RK: Constipation in the cancer patient: causes and management, in Cancer Pain: Medical Clinics of North America. Edited by Payne R, Foley KM. Philadelphia, PA, WB Saunders, 1987, pp 303–311

Portenoy R: Cancer pain: epidemiology and syndromes. Cancer 63:2298–2308, 1989

Portenoy RK: Pharmacologic approaches to the control of cancer pain. Journal of Psychosocial Oncology 8:75–107, 1990

Portenoy RK, Foley KM: Management of cancer pain, in Handbook of Psychooncology: Psychological Care of the Patient With Cancer. Edited by Holland JC, Rowland JH. New York, Oxford University, 369–382, 1989

Portenoy RK, Moulin DE, Rogers A, et al: Intravenous infusions of opioids in cancer pain: clinical review and guidelines for use. Cancer Treatment Reports 70:575–581, 1986

President's Commission for the Study of Ethical Problems in Medicine and Biomedical and Behavioral Research: Deciding to Forego Life-Sustaining

Treatment. Washington, DC, U.S. Government Printing Office, 1983

Preskorn SH, Jerkovich GS: Central nervous system toxicity of tricyclic antidepressants: phenomenology, course, risk factors, and role of therapeutic drug monitoring. J Clin Psychopharmacol 10:88–95, 1990

Quick and Painless Death Should Be a Right. New York Times, June 19, 1990, p A22

Redd W: Management of anticipatory nausea and vomiting, in Handbook of Psychooncology: Psychological Care of the Patient with Cancer. Edited by Holland JC, Rowland JH. New York, Oxford University Press, 1989, pp 423–433

Renler JB, Cooney TG: The pressure sore: pathophysiology and principles of management. Ann Intern Med 94:661–666, 1981

Saltzburg D, Breitbart W, fishman B, et al: The relationship of pain and depression to suicidal ideation in cancer patients (abstract), in Proceedings of the American Society of Clinical Oncology, Twenty-fifth Annual Meeting, San Fransico, CA, May 21–23, 1989. Philadelphia, PA, WB Saunders, American Society of Clinical Oncology, 1989, p 312

Satel SL, Nelson CJ: Stimulants in the treatment of depression: a critical overview. J Clin Psychiatry 50:241–249, 1989

Shopsin B: Bupropion: a new clinical profile in the psychobiology of depression. J Clin Psychiatry 44:140–142, 1983

Siegel K: Rational suicide: considerations for the clinician. Psychiatr Q 54:77–83, 1982

Siegel K, Tuckel P: Rational suicide and the terminally ill cancer patient. Omega 15:263–269, 1984

Silberfarb PM, Maurer LH, Cronthamel CS: Psychosocial aspects of breast cancer patients during different treatment regimens. Am J Psychiatry 137:450–455, 1980

Spiegel K, Kalb R, Pasternak G: Analgesic activity of tricyclic antidepressants. Ann Neurol 13:462–465, 1983

Stoudemire A, Fogel BS: Psychopharmacolgy in the medically ill, in Principles of Medical Psychiatry. Edited by Stoudemire A, Fogel BS. New York, Grune & Stratton, 1987, pp 79–112

Strain JJ, Liebowitz MR, Klein DF: Anxiety and panic attacks in the medically ill. Psychiatry Clin North Am 4:333–348, 1981

Tchekmedyian NS, Tait N, Moody M, et al: Appetite stimulation with megestrol acetate in cachectic cancer patients. Semin Oncol 13:37–43, 1986

Twycross RG, Lack SA: Pain relief, in Symptom Control in Far Advanced Cancer. Edited by Twycross RG, Lack SA. London, Churchill Livingston, 1983, pp 3–14

Twycross RG, Lack SA: The mouth, in Control of Alimentary Symptoms in Far Advanced Cancer. Edited by Twycross RG, Lack SA. London, Churchill

Livingston, 1986, pp 12–39

Twycross RG, Lack SA: Alimentary symptoms, in Therapeutics in Terminal Cancer. Edited by Twycross RG, Lack SA. New York, Churchill Livingston, 1990a, pp 41–79

Twycross RG, Lack SA: Respiratory symptoms, in Therapeutics in Terminal Cancer. Edited by Twycross RG, Lack SA. New York, Churchill Livingston, 1990b, pp 123–145

Twycross RG, Lack SA: Skin care, in Therapeutics in Terminal Cancer. Edited by Twycross RG, Lack SA. New York, Churchill Livingston, 1990c, pp 147–161

Walsh TD: Controlled study of imipramine and morphine in chronic pain due to cancer (abstract), in Proceedings of the American Society of Clinical Oncology Twenty-Second Annual Meeting, Los Angeles, CA, May 4–6, 1986. New York, Grune & Stratton, American Society of Clinical Oncology, 1986, p 237

Walsh T, Saunders C: Hospice care: the treatment of pain in advanced cancer. Recent Results Cancer Res 89:201–211, 1984

Woods SW, Tesar GE, Murray GB, et al: Psychostimulant treatment of depressive disorders secondary to medical illness. J Clin Psychiatry 47:12–15, 1986

World Health Organization: Cancer Pain Relief. Geneva, Switzerland, World Health Organization, 1986

Chapter 9

Management of Grief in the Cancer Setting

Harvey Max Chochinov, M.D., F.R.C.P.C.

Once he had told her something that she could not imagine: that amputees suffer pains, cramps, itches, in the leg that is no longer there. That is how she felt without him, feeling his presence where he no longer was.

Love in the Time of Cholera
Gabriel Garcìa Màrquez

*G*rief is the human emotional response to loss. For patients, families, and health care providers, the cancer setting makes confrontation with loss inescapable. Patients struggle to come to terms with the loss of their former state of good health, as well as with the anticipation of multiple losses that potentially derive from the diagnosis of cancer. Families must face the unspeakable possibility of losing a loved one. For the families of the nearly half-million Americans who will die from cancer this year alone (American Cancer Society 1989), this possibility will become a sad reality.

Health care providers face the dual obligation of providing medical care and comfort to dying patients, while guiding the family through the terminal illness (Chochinov and Holland 1989). An often overlooked aspect of this task is the difficulty of meeting the personal challenge required in coming to terms with frequent and multiple losses. In this chapter, I discuss the role of the mental health professional in each of these aspects of grieving, using clinical examples from the cancer setting.

Bereavement

Bereavement refers to the fact of loss through death. *Grief* is the feeling or affect resulting from the loss, and *mourning* is the social expression in response to loss and grief (Osterweis et al. 1984). The task of the bereaved individual can be understood from a number of theoretical perspectives. According to the psychoanalytic model, grieving requires the gradual withdrawal of "libido" from the lost object (Freud 1917). The "griefwork" is complete when the individual is able to reinvest this emotional energy into new and meaningful relationships. The interpersonal model, based on Bowlby's attachment theory (1977a, 1977b), focuses on the nature of attachment bonds and the psychosocial consequences of breaking them. Bowlby described the phenomenon of mourning as a way to try to achieve reunion with the lost person and subsequently adapt to the loss. From this derives a theory of grief that differentiates three main phases: the urge to recover the lost object, disorganization and despair, and reorganization (Bowlby 1961). Parkes (1970) later revised these phases as follows:

1. *Phase of numbness:* A stage of initial shock during which, by using various degrees of denial, the loss is partially disregarded.
2. *Phase of yearning:* The urge to recover and reunite with the deceased person predominates. Fruitless searching (e.g., scanning familiar environments for the person) results in motor restlessness, irritability, tension, and tearfulness. During this phase, it is the permanence, rather than the actual loss, that is partially disregarded.
3. *Phase of disorganization and despair:* It is during this time that attempts to recover the deceased person are given up. This phase marks acceptance of both the reality and permanence of the loss. Understandably, depression and the inability to see life as having any purpose are not uncommon.
4. *Phase of reorganization:* The bereaved individual breaks down attachments to the deceased person and begins to establish new relationships.

Worden (1982) proposed that mourning can be understood in terms of specific tasks the bereaved individual must accomplish. These include accepting the reality of the loss, experiencing the pain of grief, adjusting to an environment in which the deceased person is missing, and finally withdrawing emotional energy from the deceased person so it can be reinvested in another relationship. Regardless of one's theoretical vantage point, people tend to move from disbelief and nonacceptance to gradual acceptance of the reality and permanence of the loss. Survivors are eventually able to overcome the acutely painful and disorganizing symptoms of grief so that preoccupation with the deceased person gives way to the ability to reinvest in life and living. One must also allow for substantial individual variability: "Just as each human relationship is unique, its disruption through death will precipitate a bereavement reaction shaded by the nature and intensity of the severed bond, the life cycle stages of both the deceased and the bereft, as well as the social and cultural backdrop in the context of which the relationship began, evolved and would ultimately be mourned. Each of these will color the quality and quantity of a particular bereavement course" (Chochinov 1989; pp. 594–595).

Abnormal Grief Reactions

It is important that health care providers be taught to recognize normal grief and to differentiate it from abnormal variants. Among the best descriptions of acute grief is the work of Lindemann (1944). After the Coconut Grove Nightclub disaster in Boston, Lindemann recorded his observations of the bereaved survivors and reported the following reactions to be "pathognomonic" for grief:

1. *Somatic distress:* This occurs in waves of symptoms that include tightness in the throat, shortness of breath, a need for sighing, an empty feeling in the abdomen, lack of muscular power, and intense "tension" or "mental pain."
2. *Preoccupation with images of the deceased person:* This can include auditory, visual, or tactile hallucinations of the deceased person and illusions or misperceptions that result in "seeing" the deceased person along with a sense of unreality and increased emotional distance from others.
3. *Guilt:* The bereaved individual reviews the time before the death to find evidence of any shortcomings regarding the management of the now deceased person.
4. *Hostile reactions:* The bereaved individual may become more

irritable and easily angered, resulting in loss of warmth in relationships and the wish not to be bothered.

5. *Loss of pattern of conduct:* This often includes a diminished capacity to initiate and maintain organized patterns of activity. This may be reflected by periodic difficulties with concentration, attention, and decision making.

6. *Appearance of traits of the deceased person:* The bereaved individual may develop mannerisms and characteristics resembling those of the deceased person. In some cases, this may extend to developing symptoms of the deceased person's final illness. Lindemann (1944) emphasized that in some individuals this may herald a pathological response.

Differentiating normal grief from abnormal grief, especially from clinical depression, is often a difficult task. Unlike depression, uncomplicated bereavement does not normally present with morbid preoccupation with worthlessness, marked psychomotor retardation, or active suicidal ideation; those who are grieving also generally regard their depressed mood as a normal response. In comparing 34 depressed subjects with 34 bereaved ones, Clayton (1974) found the overlap was such as to make the two groups nondifferentiable for research purposes. A group of 109 bereaved men and women were found to have a 35% incidence of depression at 1 month; 45% of the sample population were depressed at some point during the first year, whereas 13% of the patients remained depressed throughout the entire year (Clayton et al. 1971).

Lindemann (1944) described "morbid grief reactions" as representing a distortion of normal grief. Others (e.g., DeVaul and Zisook 1976) have shown how unresolved grief can be understood in terms of arrested resolution or prolongation of any stage or symptom constellation in the normal grieving process. Although absent grief, inhibited grief, delayed grief, and abbreviated grief have all been described (Averill 1968; Parkes and Weiss 1983; Raphael 1983), chronic grief is the most common pathological variant (Parkes and Weiss 1983). It is marked by the continuous presence of symptomatology more typical of early stages of loss. Intensity does not appear to diminish over time and fails to draw to its natural conclusion. By not working through the grief, the bereaved individual is in a sense able to maintain a relationship with the deceased person.

Management Issues

It is during the terminal phase of illness that mental health professionals often have the greatest opportunity to affect the process of adaptation to loss. For the patient, this can include interventions ranging from supportive psychotherapy to more aggressive modes of treating psychiatric symptoms sometimes seen in these circumstances. Such measures can both improve the patient's quality of life and lessen the subjective distress of the family. Mental health professionals must extend their supportive stance to include family members, with particular emphasis being placed on identifying those who appear to be at risk of a complicated bereavement course. Risk factors (Table 9–1) appear to include poor social support, an ambivalent relationship to the deceased, previous psychiatric history (Vachon et al. 1982), high initial distress (Vachon 1976), multiple life crises, and a short terminal illness with little forewarning of impending death (Parkes 1975).

Most fatal outcomes due to cancer are preceded by some period of warning. This time of anticipatory grieving allows patients, loved ones, and health care providers the opportunity to prepare mentally for the impending death. Whether to reconcile differences, extend important final communications, or reaffirm feelings and wishes, this time is of vital importance and can often set the tone for the subsequent bereavement course. It is thus not surprising that sudden deaths with short advance warning have much greater impact and lasting disorganization in the life of the survivors then do deaths following adequate warning and gradual termination (Parkes 1975). The following case example illustrates a course of bereavement that began with a tragic unanticipated loss:

Table 9–1.   Risk factors for complicated bereavement

Poor social support

Ambivalent relationship to the deceased

Previous psychiatric history

High initial distress

Multiple life crises

Sudden, unanticipated death

Case 1

Ms. W, a 68-year-old woman, was referred for grief counselling 11 months after the death of her son. At the age of 39, he had been the eldest of her three children. When diagnosed with acute myelogenous leukemia, he was living in a city of considerable distance from his family. In order not to distress them prematurely, he had delayed informing his family until he was well along into his treatment. While granulocytopenic as a result of chemotherapy, he unexpectedly developed toxic shock and died. Ms. W and her husband arrived on the ward to be told their son had been taken to the intensive care unit and shortly thereafter were informed of his death.

Ms. W recalled how the following months were a nightmare during which she struggled to maintain a dominant, strong supportive role for her husband and remaining children. In anticipation of the anniversary of her son's death, however, she found herself less able to uphold this role, eventually resulting in psychiatric referral.

The initial session consisted of having Ms. W recount in as much detail as possible the events surrounding her son's death, from the first knowledge of his being ill to the final time she held his emaciated body in her arms after the failed attempt at resuscitation. Central themes included the remorse she felt in not having had the opportunity to reconcile some long-standing differences with her son, not being at his side at the time of death, and not having had the chance to say goodbye. During weekly sessions over the next 2 months, she was encouraged to express her grief in the context of an empathic therapeutic alliance. She was further educated as to the nature of grief, how symbolic connections to the deceased person (e.g., the anniversary of the death and birthdays) temporarily yet predictably intensify grief (Barton 1977), the necessity of experiencing the pain of grief, and reassurance that such pain is both normal and will become less intolerable with time.

When therapy concluded, Ms. W felt less "burdened" by her grief and able to resume numerous activities she had abandoned since her son's death, such as work and community volunteer service. Although his loss continued to be a source of sadness, she was able to think and speak of him without being overwhelmed by grief.

Mental health professionals can assist in seeing that the emotional needs of patients and families are met during the terminal phase of illness. Such needs include continuous, updated information regarding the disease status and treatment options available. This information must be delivered repeatedly and with sensitivity as to what they are currently prepared and able to hear and absorb. Families, especially, require a great deal of reassurance that they and the medical staff have done everything possible for the patient. To carry out these palliative care interventions effectively, ongoing monitoring of the patient is paramount. Even when few or no medical measures are required, the presence of the medical staff will decrease the patient's fear of abandonment, as well as establish the clinician as caring, available, and thus a potential resource for the persons soon to be bereaved. Hospital routines must be made flexible so as to accommodate the need for patient and family to spend as much time together as they deem necessary.

When possible, the family should have the opportunity to be present at the actual time of death (Engel 1964). Time alone in the room after the patient's death should be made available if the family members so desire. If an autopsy is felt to be necessary, it should be requested by the attending physician, unless another member of the medical staff has developed an especially close and supportive relationship with the family (Osterweis et al. 1984). A follow-up appointment should also be offered to discuss any findings and deal with any questions that might arise. Physicians should also review the physical and emotional symptoms that may be experienced during the grieving period. Such forewarning and reassurance of their normalcy may actually lessen their severity and any secondary anxiety about such symptoms (Osterweis et al. 1984). The following case example illustrates the importance of providing adequate psychological support for family members soon to be bereaved:

Case 2

Mr. X was a 62-year-old widower whose 22-year-old son was in the terminal phase of a central nervous system malignancy. He was extremely angry in anticipation of his son's death and projected his anger rather indiscriminately onto both medical and nursing staff. As a result of earlier psychiatric consultation for his son (which took the form of ongoing supportive psychotherapy, as well as the teaching of cognitive-behavioral techniques to manage intermittent anxiety), the psychiatric consultant had established ongoing contact with Mr. X. In the terminal phase of his son's illness, this contact consisted primarily of allowing Mr. X to ventilate his many concerns, validation of his overwhelming grief, and "gentle education" as to how his anger threatened to alienate him from much needed health care providers. Toward his son's final days, he was able to acknowledge the reality of his son's impending death and to make himself available to receiving necessary support from the health care team. On the afternoon of the day his son was later to die, he stated to the psychiatric consultant, "You know I may need you when this is all over." In saying so, he acknowledged his awareness that the door to further bereavement counselling, should it be required, was open.

The following case example poignantly illustrates many of the features that are common to grief and traces the gradual evolution of such features:

Case 3

Ms. Y, a 43-year-old nurse, was referred for grief counselling 2½ years after the death of her husband. They had known one another since their mid-teens and has been married 18 years when he was diagnosed with an inoperable central nervous system malignancy. Radiation therapy and chemotherapy did little to slow his rapid deterioration. Largely because of the efforts and determination of his wife, he was able to die at home surrounded by family, including his two preschool children.

Ms. Y was an extremely bright woman who was consciously determined to deal with her grief by "not dealing with it." Whenever she found herself experiencing pangs of loss, she would actively set out to distract herself away from them. This included using techniques equivalent to "thought stopping" and "thought substitution." Other times she desperately attempted to lose herself in work. However, by the time she presented for treatment, the very limited success of this approach was self-evident. She found herself increasingly unable to work effectively; she had never returned to sleeping in her (formerly "their") bedroom, choosing rather to sleep on the living room couch. Socially she had remained relatively inactive and admitted that periodic unavoidable reminders of her late husband left her feeling overwhelmed and fearful that she would "go crazy" if not for her ability to distract herself away from these painful thoughts.

Aside from attempts to do so in therapy, Ms. Y never spoke of her grief. During one session, while recounting the details of her husband's illness, she felt the intensity of her sense of loss "as if he had died yesterday." She further described how the physical sensation of grieving "makes the air feel thicker," thus making even the simplest of tasks more arduous.

Ms. Y's recollections always fell short of describing what actually took place on the day her husband died, claiming it to be "too painful." Two months into treatment she was able to put into words her memory of the moment he stopped breathing and her fleeting impulse, at the time, to attempt resuscitation. Although this thought was quickly dismissed, she had never been able to leave behind the guilt fed by the fantasy that, had she done so, he would have survived long enough to receive a "magical cure." This disclosure marked a turning point in therapy leading to gradual improvement. Ms. Y eventually came to understand and speak of her grief in the following way: "Grief is a toxin. While some toxins are metabolized by the liver or kidney, grief is a toxin that must be metabolized by the heart."

Impact of Grief on Staff

Health care providers who work in the cancer setting often face frequent and multiple losses of their patients. Years of medical training commonly lead to the belief that acknowledgement or expression of feelings associated with such loss is something less than "professional." Although being overwhelmed by grief can render the clinician ineffectual, the complete denial of such feeling often precludes the empathic stance necessary to meet the emotional needs of bereaved family members. Either extreme may be an indicator that the clinician's mental health is at risk. The following case example illustrates the emotional aftermath seen among oncology staff after the death of a patient:

Case 4

Ms. Z was 22 years old when she died in the hospital from Hodgkin's disease. She was a bright, warm, human being who had endeared herself to both nursing and medical staff. Her youth, sensitivity, and humor (even in the face of personal tragedy) made her death an especially painful one for all staff involved in her care. Shortly thereafter, a "psychosocial round" was held for the oncology staff to specifically discuss Ms. Z and the personal impact of her loss. (These meetings take place weekly to explore a variety of psychosocial issues in oncology; they are chaired by the psychiatric consultant and provide a forum for mutual support [Chochinov et al. 1987].)

Whereas some staff members shared fond memories of Ms. Z, others expressed concern and anger regarding some specific aggressive and invasive measures taken during her final days. Some voiced self-doubt as to whether they personally might have done more. The group was able to share their sense of loss and impotence, while also managing to offer support to individual members.

Although this meeting did not end the process of grieving (nor was it intended to), it did allow for the expression of feelings associated with Ms. Z's death, validate the legitimacy of such feelings, and underline the need to mourn. It also strongly reinforced the notion that a sense of loss is to be expected after the death of a patient and that mourning such losses is not "unprofessional."

Summary

Loss is ubiquitous in the cancer setting. As a result, the role and activities of mental health care professionals who work in this area will cover an enormous range. For patients, this can mean enhancement of palliative care services and improved quality of life. Families may benefit from emotional guidance through the terminal phase of illness along with bereavement counselling for those in need. Finally, such activities should include a component directed toward maintaining the mental health of health care providers who choose to work in this emotionally demanding area.

References

American Cancer Society: Cancer Facts and Figures. New York, American Cancer Society, 1989

Averill JR: Grief: its nature and significance. Psychol Bull 70:721–748, 1968

Barton D: Dying and Death: A Clinical Guide for Caregivers. Baltimore, MD, Williams & Wilkins, 1977

Bowlby J: Process of mourning. Int J Psychoanal 42:317–340, 1961

Bowlby J: The making and breaking of affectional bonds, I: aetiology and psychopathology in the light of attachment theory. Br J Psychiatry 130:201–210, 1977a

Bowlby J: The making and breaking of affectional bonds, II: some principles of psychotherapy. Br J Psychiatry 130:421–431, 1977b

Chochinov HM: Bereavement: a review for oncology health professionals. Cancer Invest 7:593–600, 1989

Chochinov HM, Holland JC: Bereavement: special issues in oncology, in Handbook of Psychooncology: Psychological Care of the Patient With Cancer. Edited by Holland JC, Rowland JH. New York, Oxford University Press, 1989, pp 612–627

Chochinov HM, Breitbart W, Brish M, et al: Psychosocial Support Groups on a Neuro-Oncology Unit: Current Concepts in Psycho-Oncology and AIDS (syllabus of the postgraduate course). New York, Memorial Sloan-Kettering Cancer Center, 1987

Clayton P: Mourning and depression: their similarities and differences. Can J Psychiatry 1:309–312, 1974

Clayton P, Halikes JA, Maurice WI: The bereavement of the widowed. Diseases of the Nervous System 32:597–604, 1971

DeVaul R, Zisook S: Unresolved grief: clinical considerations. Postgrad Med 59:267–271, 1976

Engel GL: Grief and grieving. Am J Nurs 64:93–98, 1964

Freud S: Mourning and melancholia (1917), in Standard Edition of the Complete Psychological Works of Sigmund Freud, Vol 14. Translated and edited by Strachey J. New York, WW Norton, 1963, pp 243–258

Lindemann E: Symptomatology and management of acute grief. Am J Psychiatry 101:141–148, 1944

Osterweis M, Solomon F, Green M (eds): Bereavement: Reactions Consequences and Care. Washington, DC, National Academy Press, 1984

Parkes CM: Seeking and finding a lost object: evidence from recent studies of the reaction to bereavement. Soc Sci Med 4:181–201, 1970

Parkes CM: Determinants of outcome following bereavement. Omega 6:303–323, 1975

Parkes CM, Weiss R: Recovery From Bereavement. New York, Basic Books, 1983

Raphael B: The Anatomy of Bereavement. New York, Basic Books, 1983

Vachon MLS: Grief and bereavement following the death of a spouse. Canadian Psychiatric Association Journal 21:35–44, 1976

Vachon MLS, Sheldon AR, Lancee WJ, et al: Predictors and correlates of high distress in adaptation to conjugal bereavement. Am J Psychiatry 139:998–1002, 1982

Worden W: Grief Counselling and Grief Therapy: A Handbook for the Mental Health Practitioner. New York, Springer, 1982

Chapter 10

The Stress of Caring for Cancer Patients

Kathryn M. Kash, Ph.D.
William Breitbart, M.D.

*T*hose of us who work intensively with cancer patients have chosen a rewarding but stressful occupation. Researchers have identified the stressors encountered by physicians and nurses who work in the oncology setting (Chiriboga et al. 1983; Fox 1962; Gentry and Parkes 1982; Mount 1986; Moynihan and Outlaw 1984; Peteet et al. 1989; Schmale et al. 1987; Spikes and Holland 1975; Vachon 1987; Yasko 1983), the consequences of such stress (Hall et al. 1979; Holland and Holland 1985; Lederberg 1989; Maslach 1979; Mount 1986), and factors that play a role in adaptive coping with such stress (Hartl 1979; Kobasa 1979; Kobasa and Puccetti 1983; Koocher 1979; Mount 1986). Staff stress researchers have not, however, adequately addressed these issues as they relate to mental health professionals who work with cancer patients.

Wise (1981) described the burnout syndrome in consultation-liaison psychiatrists working on general medical and surgical units. Holland (1989) described the stresses on mental health professionals working in oncology, based on her experiences and those of her psychiatric colleagues and trainees over a 10-year period at Memorial Sloan-Kettering Cancer Center. No empirical studies using the "stress" or "burnout" models have been conducted with mental health professionals in the oncology setting. However, descriptive and experiential reports in the literature, such as those cited above and those that deal with countertransference issues in the psychotherapy of cancer patients (Klagsburn 1983; Massie et al. 1989; Sourkes 1982; Spikes and Holland 1975), form the basis of our current understanding of the stresses encountered by therapists caring for cancer patients.

In this chapter, we review the major sources of stress for staff in a cancer setting, the consequences of stress, and strategies for decreasing the deleterious effects of stress, thus improving morale and performance. We also highlight the unique stressors on mental health professionals and the important role that psychiatrists play in staff stress interventions.

Stressors on Mental Health Professionals

The psychiatrist, psychologist, social worker, or psychiatric nurse engaged in work with cancer patients is subject to many of the same stressors encountered by the oncology staff (as described below). There are, however, unique stressors that confront the mental health professional in the cancer setting (Table 10–1). The most salient include the nature of psychotherapy with cancer patients, countertransference issues, and work or role-related stressors.

Nature of Psychotherapy in Cancer

The unique nature of psychotherapy in the cancer setting is a source of stress, especially for those whose training has not exposed them to work with the medically ill. Psychotherapy with cancer patients demands a far more active stance and use of the self than is true of traditional psychotherapy, making the need for self-awareness more important (Massie et al. 1989). The therapist in the oncology setting must be knowledgeable not only about psychotherapeutic techniques, but also about cancer and cancer treatment (Klagsburn 1983). He or she must be familiar with the principles of crisis intervention, supportive psychotherapy, family therapy, liaison psychiatry, and cognitive-behavioral techniques.

Enormous "flexibility" as to scheduling of times for therapy and the setting in which psychotherapy takes place is required. Patients miss appointments due to illness, and psychotherapy often takes place in a hospital room or even an intensive care unit. In addition, the psychotherapist is constantly confronted with issues of death and dying. Perhaps more than any other member of the oncology staff, it is the therapist who engages the patient in an exploration of concerns and feelings about death and grief. Introspection about one's own vulnerability helps reduce personalized responses by psychotherapists (Massie

Table 10–1. Stressors on mental health professionals

1. Nature of psychotherapy in cancer
   Countertransference issues
   Issues of death and loss

2. Isolation from collegial peers
   Few "psychooncologists"
   Lack of peer support
   Unique specialty

3. Ambiguity of role
   Undefined role
   Competing roles
   "Consultation" role

4. Absence of a "tool"
   Helplessness
   Specific skills

5. Response of medical colleagues
   Ambivalence toward psychiatry
   Professional credibility

6. Low status of psychosocial issues
   "Curing" cancer more important
   "Real" medicine more compelling

7. Dealing with the sense of urgency
   Life and death issues
   Crisis situations

8. Solving insolvable problems
   "Fix it"—quickly
   Unrealistic expectations

9. Work conditions
   Difficult to schedule hours
   Work load
   Lack of privacy

10. Systems problems
    Hospital as a social system
    Work with staff

11. Fears of cancer
    "Cancerphobia"
    Phases of emotional reactions

Adapted from Holland JC: "Stresses on the Mental Health Professional," in *Handbook of Psychooncology: Psychological Care of the Patient With Cancer.* Edited by Holland JC, Rowland JH. New York, Oxford University Press, 1989, pp. 678–682.

et al. 1989; Sourkes 1982). Insight into personal views of death and the ability to deal with death and losses are useful as well.

Countertransference Issues

Countertransference reactions occur commonly in psychotherapy; however, psychotherapy with cancer patients tends to elicit some common countertransference reactions that should be well known to therapists engaging in this work. **The first is the need to try to "save" patients from their cancer illness or death.** The therapist may wish to rescue patients from their dreadful plight. Unfortunately, disease often progresses, and failure to save or rescue patients provokes feelings of helplessness and impotence, as well as a sense of futility. Low self-esteem and depression may result and sometimes lead to a sense of resentment toward patients. In an attempt to deal with these feelings of helplessness and futility, the therapist may become overinvolved in the patients' medical care, encouraging or demanding inappropriately aggressive or unrealistic interventions.

Staff members, including mental health professionals, often find the transition from active treatment to palliative care difficult. Accepting altered treatment goals and relinquishing the hope of survival for a special patient can be very painful (Spikes and Holland 1975). Inability to recognize that such a transition in care is necessary can lead to a delay in dealing with practical issues, such as do-not-resuscitate (DNR) orders. Unaware of such countertransference reactions, a psychiatrist working with a cancer patient may develop an adversarial relationship with other health professionals involved in that individual's care. A grandiose or self-serving attitude may develop whereby the psychotherapist feels that only he or she understands the patient and knows how best to care for him or her medically. Unchecked, such attitudes can lead to staff conflict. More commonly such an attitude reflects an overinflated sense of responsibility for the patient's fate, which can result in enormous guilt once the patient's condition ultimately worsens. An alternative response to feelings of helplessness and futility involves avoidance of the patient or premature withdrawal from the patient. Such avoidance or withdrawal is often based on unrecognized angry feelings that reflect the impotence felt in dealing with a patient whose condition progresses and deteriorates despite all efforts (Massie et al. 1989).

The second common countertransference reaction is the need to "protect" the patient. This often involves not confronting or bringing up for discussion, even when appropriate, topics that may be painful or emotionally distressing for the patient. Consequently, important issues may go unaddressed such as the patient's feelings about pain, suffering, and death and practical issues such as a will, DNR status, and tying up financial loose ends. It is also important for the psychiatrist to confront extreme denial and other maladaptive defenses on the part of the patient, especially when they interfere with treatment compliance. Recognition of our human limitations and personal vulnerabilities to loss are as important as being aware of these common countertransference reactions. Hopefully, such awareness can benefit our patients, colleagues, and ourselves.

Work- and Role-Related Stressors

With the exception of the relatively few specialized settings, such as Memorial Sloan-Kettering Cancer Center, the mental health professional who provides psychological services to cancer patients is isolated from collegial peers. Psychooncology is a relatively new field, and the psychiatrist with an interest in the psychological care of cancer patients may find that he or she is the only such individual in a particular institution. The lack of peer support or peer supervision from other mental health professionals adds to the stress of such work. Such isolation, combined with the limitations of the consultant role, leads to feelings of being an outsider working with "someone else's patients." Attempts to integrate into the oncology setting often highlight the fact that expectations of what a mental health professional's role will be are rather idiosyncratic and often undefined. Occasionally there may be several members of other disciplines whose job it is to provide psychosocial services. Conflicts arising from such competitive situations can be minimized with definition of roles and division of labor in a cooperative fashion. Role definition can develop as a function of special skills. Psychiatrists may focus on psychiatric assessment and pharmacotherapy, whereas a nurse or social worker may concentrate efforts in providing family or group counseling and teaching relaxation techniques.

In a cancer setting, psychosocial issues often take a back seat to exciting medical and oncological issues that seem somehow more compelling to medical staff. This low status of psychosocial issues is further compounded by our medical colleagues' ambivalence toward psychiatry. Medical staff often do not value or appreciate what mental health professionals can offer in the cancer setting. This does not, however, prevent them from calling us to solve insolvable problems or "fix" difficult patients or situations that are not correctable. The psychiatrist may feel compelled to make recommendations prematurely in an attempt to deal with crisis situations that arise with a sense of urgency.

Unexpected medical crises make keeping a schedule of hours to see patients quite difficult. Emergency consultations may require evaluating a patient in the late evening, sometimes in a setting that lacks privacy. Often the issues involved present ethical dilemmas that have life-or-death consequences and may involve the patient, their family, multiple levels of medical staff, and hospital administration. With a number of difficult and complex cases, and no colleagues to share the work load, fatigue and stress set in.

The initial phases of psychiatric work in oncology are accompanied by some predictable emotional reactions. Transient "cancerphobia" is somewhat universal among those who are new to the cancer unit. An initial period of numbness leads into anxious and then depressed feelings after a period of 3 months, when the burden of frequent patient deaths is felt. Eventually a sense of resolution allows for an evaluation of the rewards of this work versus its stresses. Those who keep at it beyond a year usually stay in the field (Holland 1989).

Stressors Specific to the Cancer Setting

Compared with general medical settings, the cancer unit has a set of specific stressors (Table 10–2) that make working with cancer patients challenging. The nature of cancer and cancer treatment, difficult ethical dilemmas in treatment decision making, emotional reactions of patients and staff to cancer, and poor staff communication or conflict all contribute to the stressful cancer work environment. By virtue of the fact that mental health professionals are part of the treatment team, along with oncologists and oncology nurses, they are subject to many of the same work-related stressors.

Vachon (1987) described the stressors that are regularly encountered by oncologists and oncology nurses. These include caring for the patient who is extremely ill, dealing with the deaths of patients of all

ages, poor staff communications, being intensely involved with patients and their families, conflicts between research and clinical care
goals, and the work load imposed by the complicated and taxing work
of palliative care. The gravity of the illness under treatment and the
emphasis on clinical investigation in the cancer center make the modern treatment setting comparable to the social environment of the
metabolic ward described so elegantly by Fox (1962) almost three

Table 10–2. Stressors specific to the cancer setting

1. Nature of cancer
    High morbidity and mortality
    Confronting death
2. Nature of cancer treatment
    Lack of efficacy
    Side effects
    Inflicting pain and/or disfigurement
    Complex technology
    Palliative treatment
3. Treatment decision making
    Terminal care decisions
    Do-not-resuscitate (DNR) orders
    Surrogate decision making
    Third-party conflicts
    Ethical issues
4. Patient reactions to cancer
    Unrealistic expectations
    Projected anger
    Grief, depression
    Suicidal ideation
    Requests for euthanasia (assisted suicide)
5. Staff reactions to cancer
    Cancer "phobia"
    Powerlessness
6. Interstaff conflicts
    Disagreements on appropriateness of interventions
    Enormous work load
    Conflict between clinical and research responsibilities
7. Isolation outside of work place
    Provokes anxiety in others
    "Isn't it depressing?"
    "You're a saint!"

decades ago when the initial use of steroids for otherwise fatal diseases was being studied. The same problems of dealing with uncertainty, frustration with failure, and sadness when patients die of their disease face us today. Having significant success at work, feeling one is in the right field, seeing some patients getting better and going home, and being complimented for a professional job well done contribute to an increased sense of accomplishment. However, seeing several patients die in a short period of time, treating patients of one's own age, or losing a patient one is close with all take their toll on oncologists and oncology nurses.

Trust and communication between patients and staff, as well as between staff members, are of the utmost importance for the emotional well-being of the patient and cohesiveness of the staff. This is crucial in advanced stages of cancer when it becomes necessary to discuss painful realities, including appropriateness of DNR orders. Communication with patients around these issues are particularly stressful. Mount (1986) described this difficult issue in the care of cancer patients when the decision must be made to change from active treatment of disease to palliation and comfort. This transition and the decisions that follow (e.g., the DNR order) are among the most painful aspects of oncology. These decisions are the most frequent cause of conflict among staff, and with family members, because the views are so intertwined with personal values and beliefs.

Schmale et al. (1987) conducted a stress survey on 147 physicians who were members of the American Society of Clinical Oncology. The physicians felt challenged by oncology. Nevertheless, they felt pressured and suffered from the negative responses and emotional problems of patients and families, the burden of dealing with dying patients, the frustration of ineffective treatments, and the impact of negative personal life events. They identified a need for more emotional support for themselves as well as their patients. In a study done at Dana-Farber Cancer Institute (Peteet et al. 1989), the greatest source of stress for physicians was their inability to help patients. Nurses felt that ethical issues, particularly as they revolve around DNR status and competing research and clinical goals, were the most stressful.

The studies on stress associated with the practice of cancer nursing indicate that oncology nurses are particularly vulnerable to the effects of stress. The stressors for the oncology nurse are multidimensional and arise from a complex interplay of organizational, situational, and personal variables (Yasko 1983). The nursing care requirements of a cancer patient become increasingly more complex as the patient's illness progresses and functional status diminishes. Specific stressors for the nurse include the negotiation of differing perceptions of the disease held by "patient and family" and by "patient and physician"; technologically complex patient care requirements; interpersonal communication problems; and limited institutional support (Chiriboga et al. 1983; Gentry and Parkes 1982; Moynihan and Outlaw 1984).

It is also important to take into account the inevitability of personal losses, illnesses, and conflicts, at times coinciding with work stressors. Having family members ill or diagnosed as having cancer makes it difficult for professionals to deal with their patients without overidentification. Having interpersonal, family, or financial problems increases the stress placed on an individual and can increase the amount of emotional distress. In addition, having personality traits that lead to overinvolvement at work and little time for avocational activities may leave the professional isolated from family members and friends. These sources of stress for oncologists and oncology nurses have both personal and professional consequences.

Consequences of Stress

The consequences of stress in the cancer setting include the development of physical symptoms, psychological symptoms, "burnout," and even more serious psychiatric impairment (e.g., alcoholism, drug abuse, or depression). The most frequent physical symptoms of chronic stress include tension headache, exhaustion, fatigue, insomnia, gastrointestinal disturbances (with increase or decrease in appetite) when no medical explanation can be found, and minor aches and pains (often questioned as signs of leukemia or cancer). In a study (Kash and Holland 1990) conducted at Memorial Sloan-Kettering Cancer Center, physicians and nurses with more family stressors reported more physical symptoms than those with fewer family stressors. These findings were similar to those of Ullrich and Fitzgerald (1990) who found that interpersonal difficulties were related to physical symptoms among nurses in a cancer setting.

Often accompanying such physical symptoms are signs of psychological distress (Table 10–3). Psychological symptoms of stress in cancer staff include loss of enthusiasm for work, depression, irritability and frustration, and a cynical view of medicine and colleagues (Hall et al. 1979; Holland and Holland 1985; Maslach 1979; Mount 1986). Physicians and nurses can become overinvolved in their work, with excessive dedication and commitment, longer hours with less productivity, and decreased sensitivity to the emotional needs of patients and others; conversely they may become detached and disinterested in medical practice. These two presentations of "burnout" in oncologists and oncology nurses have been described as the "I must do everything" syndrome and the "I hate medicine" syndrome. Potential outcomes of both of these two syndromes, if allowed to progress, include alcoholism, substance abuse, depression, and even suicide (Hall et al. 1979; Holland and Holland 1985; Mount 1986).

The burnout syndrome, described by Maslach (1979), is characterized by emotional exhaustion, depersonalization, and lack of a sense of personal accomplishment. Emotional exhaustion is experienced as being emotionally overextended and exhausted by work. *Depersonalization* is a poor term to describe the sense of distance and reduced empathy that the person usually feels toward patients. Lack of personal accomplishment is expressed by comments such as "What do I ever accomplish anyway?" Staff begin to feel that all treatment is futile in cancer, so why bother at all. Millerd (1977) conceptualized these problems as a form of survivor syndrome, like posttraumatic stress disorder, in health caregivers who have dealt repeatedly with losses from death; some of the adverse symptoms are the same as those seen in survivors of natural disasters.

Table 10–3. Psychological symptoms of stress in physicians and nurses

---

No enthusiasm for work

Hard to get up to go to work

Mood characterized by depression, tension, irritability, and/or easy frustration

Detachment characterized by cynicism, negativity, "why bother," tuned out, shortening hours, or feeling less responsible about obligations

Overinvolvement characterized by feelings that "nobody can do it right but me," feelings that "nobody works but me," working longer hours with less productivity, or taking work home

---

In a study conducted at Memorial Sloan-Kettering Cancer Center, "burnout" was examined in house staff (interns and residents) and nurses (Kash and Holland 1990). Interesting gender differences emerged regarding burnout, especially as related to emotional exhaustion and depersonalization. Women (interns, residents, and nurses) were more emotionally exhausted and more depersonalized than were men (interns, residents, and nurses). Interns were more emotionally exhausted and more depersonalized than residents or nurses regardless of gender. However, being religious (even a little bit) and having a hardy personality were factors that predicted less emotional exhaustion. Negative work stressors, such as inequitable work loads, multiple patient deaths, or conflict with other staff members, all lead to greater burnout.

As symptoms of burnout progress from mild to severe, there is an inability to function, and depression may result. Alcohol and drug use may become a form of coping. The more serious consequences of stress occur when the early signs and symptoms of burnout are ignored or denied by the physician or nurse (and colleagues and family). Typically, physicians or nurses will deny the existence of a problem with depression or alcohol or drug use and delay seeking help. Fears of stigmatization, as well as legitimate concerns regarding professional licensure restrictions, make it difficult for doctors or nurses to seek psychiatric treatment for depression or drug use.

Coping With Stress

There is an interaction between individual and environmental variables that results in a range of ways of coping and adapting to stress. There are both personal (personality type and coping style) and interpersonal (social support and support of the work environment) resources available to counter professional stressors.

An effort to reinforce certain personality characteristics that lead to better coping with stressful situations is one approach to reducing stress. Kobasa (1979) described the "hardy" personality that copes well in stressful environments and is characterized by commitment, control, and challenge. The combination of a sense of commitment to oneself and the various areas in life including work, an attitude that one has influence or control over what occurs, and a sense of being challenged in the face of a changing environment have been shown, when present, to be associated with fewer mental and physical symptoms of stress. Hardiness is said to lead to a perception, interpretation, and handling of stressful events that prevent excessive activation of arousal and therefore result in fewer symptoms of stress.

Empirical research has found that business executives, lawyers, army officers, and others professionals with a high number of stresses who had a strong sense of commitment to self and work, a more positive attitude toward change, and a greater belief in control over life reported fewer physical symptoms than those who did not have this personality style (Kobasa 1979; Kobasa and Puccetti 1983). These were all professional groups that are similar to physicians in socioeconomic status. Preliminary findings from studies of physicians and nurses at Memorial Sloan-Kettering Cancer Center suggest that being "hardy" helps in coping with the stress of working in a cancer center. High levels of hardiness were a significant predictor of less burnout, less demoralization, and fewer physical symptoms (Kash and Holland 1990).

A variety of coping methods can be introduced on both the personal level and the organizational level and can be useful in the prevention and management of burnout (Table 10–4) (Hartl 1979; Koocher 1979; Mount 1986). One of the most important strategies is to be able to recognize the physical and psychological symptoms of stress in oneself. It is additionally important to identify them in colleagues and point out that such symptoms are common, transient, and reversible when dealt with early. Discomfort in pointing out emotional distress in a colleague should not be any greater than suggesting a consultation for a medical symptom. In the cancer center, having support from one's peers helps decrease feelings of demoralization (Kash and Holland 1990).

Oncologists and nurses who take a positive attitude toward themselves and their work deal better with stress. Daily challenges are less overwhelming. Maintaining self-esteem and self-confidence, often shaken when caring for cancer patients, is helpful and contributes to communication characterized by mutual respect. Maintaining a sense of humor (through the use of black or gallows humor) allows laughing at tragedy as a way to lighten the situation. It is sometimes poorly understood by others who see it as disrespectful. It is actually an important coping device that, when shared with close colleagues, contributes to the esprit de corps. The "M*A*S*H" mentality evidenced by the familiar Korean War film of surgeons in a field hospital portrays its use extremely well.

There are several other methods that physicians and nurses use to help them cope and relax (Table 10–5). Interestingly, in a study at Memorial Sloan-Kettering Cancer Center (Kash and Holland 1990), all groups queried used talking to someone they know, humor, watching television, and eating or drinking coffee as the four most common ways to cope with stress. In addition, exercise and diet have been found useful by our staff. Exercise, particularly if practiced on a regular basis, reduces stress symptoms. Adequate sleep prevents the associated problems of fatigue and irritability. Change of pace by taking breaks and vacations is important; the fresh look at work problems that comes after time away confirms its value. Attention to an avocation ensures a change of pace and, when it entails vigorous physical exercise, helps relieve frustration and physical symptoms of stress. Relaxation is another way to cope with symptoms of stress. Meditation, yoga, biofeedback, and progressive relaxation work well. Consistency in using relaxation is the key to making it work.

Mental health professionals, subject to many of the same stressors as oncologists and oncology nurses, can obviously use and benefit from many of these coping methods. Several important measures that may facilitate a mental health professional's adjustment to working with cancer patients have been suggested by Holland (1989). Psychiatrists beginning to work in the oncology setting must be oriented to the succession of emotions they may feel (i.e., increased fears of cancer, anxiety, depression, and adaption). They must also receive formal

Table 10–4. Coping strategies

Recognize and monitor symptoms

Change pace and balance diet

Decrease overtime

Exercise

Maintain sense of humor

Seek consultation if symptoms are severe

Discuss work-related stresses with others who share the same problems

Visit counterpart in other institutions; look for new solutions to problems

Note stress symptoms in colleagues and discuss with them; suggest referral, if needed

instruction in oncology, becoming familiar with types of cancer, treatments, and prognoses associated with each. Integration into a cancer unit by allocating time to a single group enhances the sense of belonging. Using a liaison model to a particular unit (bone marrow transplant unit or neurooncology unit), or service (pain service or rehabilitation service) allows more personal interaction with staff members who then better utilize the mental health professional's services. Having such a liaison relationship allows for the opportunity to teach about psychosocial aspects of cancer, to learn about issues related to specific areas of cancer, and to develop research hypotheses.

Table 10–5. Most and least used ways of coping or relaxing by nurses and doctors

House staff (*n* = 76)	Attendings (*n* = 35)	Alumni (*n* = 68)	Nurses (*n* = 82)
1. Talk to someone	Humor	Humor	Talk to someone
2. Humor	Talk to someone	Eating or drinking coffee	Humor
3. Television	Television	Talk to someone	Eating or drinking coffee
4. Eating or drinking coffee	Exercise	Television	Television
13. Prayer or meditation	Prayer or meditation	Prayer or meditation	Aspirin
14. Relaxation activities	Smoke	Relaxation activities	Smoke
15. Smoke	Medication	Medication	Relaxation activities
16. Medication	Relaxation activities	Smoke	Medication

Source. Adapted from Kash KM, Holland JC: "Reducing Stress in Medical Oncology House Officers: A Preliminay Report of a Prospective Intervention Study," in *Educating Competent and Humane Physicians.* Edited by Hendrie HC, Lloyd C. Bloomington, IN, Indiana University Press, 1990, pp. 183–195.

Organizing teaching materials, lectures, and research studies gives the psychiatrist or other mental health professional a sense of professional identity. A research orientation or perspective allows the mental health practitioner to view painful and emotional issues in a different way. The research model is also a means of enhancing collegiality and collaboration with oncological peers. The need for peer support is critical. Often the psychooncologist is isolated from psychiatric peers and lacks that critical mass of psychosocial practitioners that helps provide mutual support. On a practical level, one may want to insist on having a core of psychosocial professionals when beginning a psychooncology service. One also, however, can find support through collaborations with colleagues at other cancer centers or through the activities of professional organizations such as the American Society of Psychiatric Oncology/AIDS (ASPOA). Ultimately, the mental health professional must be aware of the stresses of cancer work and recognize the need for patience, humor, and the support of others.

Interventions to Reduce Stress: Mental Health Professionals' Role in Staff Support

Mental health professionals can perform several staff support roles in the oncology setting. Lederberg (1989) categorized these roles into 1) support and backup to unit leaders and 2) facilitator of communications. Fulfilling such roles can be accomplished with activities that range from providing support to colleagues or helping identify and deal with troubled staff to leading groups and conferences or participating in daily rounds. Ideally, an active role on the unit makes the liaison psychiatrist most familiar with the problems of the unit. The mental health consultant can be an outsider, but this usually limits his or her effectiveness.

There is a great need to find ways to help oncology staff cope with stress as it relates to the cancer environment. In addition to coping strategies that can be used on a personal level, organizational and supportive measures can be undertaken to assist oncology staff in the adaptation to clinical care in oncology. Below we describe such an intervention model designed and carried out by a collaboration between psychiatrists, psychologists, psychiatric nurses, oncologists, and oncology nurses (Kash and Holland 1990).

At Memorial Sloan-Kettering Cancer Center, the psychiatry team used a supportive intervention model to reduce the stressors on house staff and nurses through enhanced information, communication, sense of cohesiveness, and support. This intervention increased the staff's sense of control, commitment, and challenge at work, thereby reducing the physical and psychological symptoms of stress and avoiding negative impact on patient care. There were several components to this model: orientation for new house staff and nurses; a weekly meeting with house staff and nurses to listen to their "gripes" at a "pizza lunch"; a weekly interdisciplinary unit meeting—the collaborative practice meeting—that explored patient and staff issues and attempted to identify problems and seek resolutions; and daily interdisciplinary rounds with the staff (including psychiatrists) involved in patient care. A liaison psychiatrist was an active participant in each component of this intervention model.

The results of this year-long educational and supportive intervention, as compared with a control unit, indicated that it was significantly ($P < .01$) effective in reducing the burnout of residents (Kash and Holland 1990). The impact was less obvious for interns and nurses, perhaps because of their greater levels of stress for which the intervention was not powerful enough to show an impact. For all subjects in the study, it was clear that those who had a hardy personality style had less burnout and psychological distress. One of the most important findings was that patients expressed greater satisfaction with the "art" of their medical care (e.g., interest, sensitivity, and compassion from the staff) on the intervention unit than did patients on the control floor. Thus one could conclude that increased sensitivity, support, and communication for the staff members also increased the patients' positive perception of the "human" side of care.

Summary

Working in a cancer center is stressful for oncologists, oncology nurses, and mental health professionals who are committed to caring for cancer patients. Although there are many factors, both personal and work related, that contribute to "burnout," there are methods of coping with such stress that allow those of us who work in the cancer setting to appreciate and enjoy the rewards of cancer care. Recognizing our limitations and developing a supportive work environment are important parts of a strategy for stress management that hopefully will allow us to continue doing this difficult but vitally necessary work: the work of caring for the cancer patient.

References

Chiriboga D, Jenkins G, Baily J: Stress and coping among hospice nurses: test of analytic model. Nurs Res 32:294–299, 1983

Fox R: Experiment Perilous. Glencoe, IL, Free Press, 1962

Gentry ED, Parkes KR: Psychologic stress in intensive care unit and nonintensive care unit nurses: a review of the past decade. Heart Lung 4:43–47, 1982

Hall RCW, Gardner ER, Perl M, et al: The professional burnout syndrome. Psychiatric Opinion 16:12–17, 1979

Hartl DE: Stress management and the nurse, in Stress Management. Edited by Sutterley DC, Donnelly GF. Germantown, MD, Aspen, 1979, pp 163–172

Holland JC: Stresses on the mental health professional, in Handbook of Psychooncology: Psychological Care of the Patient With Cancer. Edited by Holland JC, Rowland JH. New York, Oxford University Press, 1989, pp 678–682

Holland JC, Holland JF: A neglected problem: the stresses of cancer care on physicians. Primary Care and Cancer 5:16–22, 1985

Kash KM, Holland JC: Reducing stress in medical oncology house officers: a preliminary report of a prospective intervention study, in Educating Competent and Humane Physicians. Edited Hendrie HC, Lloyd C. Bloomington, IN, Indiana University Press, 1990, pp 183–195

Klagsburn S: The making of a cancer psychotherapist. Journal of Psychosocial Oncology 1:55–60, 1983

Kobasa SC: Stressful life events, personality, and health: an inquiry into hardiness. J Pers Soc Psychol 37:1–11, 1979

Kobasa SC, Puccetti MC: Personality and social resources in stress resistence. J Pers Soc Psychol 45:839–850, 1983

Koocher GP: Adjustment and coping strategies among the caretakers of cancer patients. Soc Work Health Care 5:145–150, 1979

Lederberg M: Psychological problems of staff and their management, in Handbook of Psychooncology: Psychological Care of the Patient With Cancer. Edited by Holland JC, Rowland JH. New York, Oxford University Press, 1989, pp 678–682

Maslach C: The burnout syndrome and patient care, in Stress and Survival: The Emotional Realities of Life-Threatening Illness. Edited by Garfield CA. St. Louis, MO, Mosby, 1979, pp 89–96

Massie MJ, Holland JC, Straker N: Psychotherapeutic Interventions, in Handbook of Psychooncology: Psychological Care of the Patient With Cancer.

Edited by Holland JC, Rowland JH. New York, Oxford University Press, 1989, pp 455–469

Millerd EJ: Health professionals as survivors. Journal of Psychiatric Nursing and Mental Health Services 15:33–36, 1977

Mount BM: Dealing with our losses. J Clin Oncol 4:1127–1134, 1986

Moynihan RT, Outlaw E: Nursing support groups in a cancer center. Journal of Psychosocial Oncology 2:33–48, 1984

Peteet JR, Murrary-Ross D, Medeiros C, et al: Job stress and satisfaction among the staff members at a cancer center. Cancer 64:975–982, 1989

Schmale J, Weinberg N, Pieper S: Satisfactions, stresses, and coping mechanisms of oncologists in clinical practice (abstract). Proceedings of the American Society of Clinical Oncology 6:255, 1987

Sourkes BM: The Deepening Shade: Psychological Aspects of Life-Threatening Illness. Pittsburgh, PA, University of Pittsburgh Press, 1982

Spikes J, Holland J: The physician's response to the dying patient, in Psychological Care of the Medically Ill. Edited by Strain JJ, Grossman S. New York, Appleton-Century-Crofts, 1975, pp 138–148

Ullrich A, Fitzgerald P: Stress experienced by physicians and nurses in the cancer ward. Soc Sci Med 31:1013–1022, 1990

Vachon MLS: Occupational Stress in the Care of the Critically Ill, the Dying, and the Bereaved. Washington, DC, Hemisphere, 1987

Wise TN: Burnout: stresses in consultation-liaison psychiatry. Psychosomatics 22:744–751, 1981

Yasko JM: Variables which predict burnout experienced by oncology nurse specialsits. Cancer Nurs 6:109–116, 1983

Index

---

*Page numbers printed in **boldface** type refer to tables or figures.*